THE CANCER AT

Also published by the
American Cancer Society:

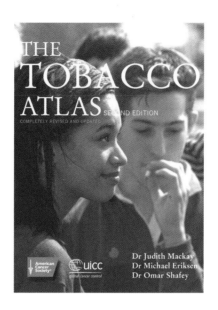

THE CANCER ATLAS

Dr Judith Mackay
Dr Ahmedin Jemal
Dr Nancy C Lee
Dr D Maxwell Parkin

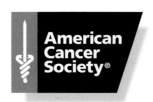

Published by the American Cancer Society
1599 Clifton Road NE
Atlanta, Georgia 30329, USA
www.cancer.org

1 3 5 7 9 10 8 6 4 2

ISBN 0-944235-62-X

Library of Congress Cataloguing-in-Publication Data
The Cancer Atlas / Judith Mackay...[et al.]
p. ; cm.
Includes bibliographical references and index.
ISBN 0-944235-62-X (paperback)
1. Cancer Atlases. 2. Cancer Epidemiology.
[DNLM: 1. Neoplasms-epidemiology-Atlases. QZ 17 C215 2006]
I. Mackay, Judith. II. American Cancer Society.
RC262.C274 2006
614.5'999-dc22
2006040672

Produced for the American Cancer Society by
Myriad Editions Limited
6–7 Old Steine, Brighton BN1 1EJ, UK
www.MyriadEditions.com

Edited and co-ordinated for Myriad Editions by
Candida Lacey, Jannet King and Sadie Mayne
Design and graphics by Corinne Pearlman and Isabelle Lewis
Maps created by Isabelle Lewis

Printed on paper produced from sustainable sources.
Printed and bound in Hong Kong through Phoenix Offset Limited
under the supervision of Bob Cassels, The Hanway Press, London

CONTENTS

Part One: INTRODUCTION

Part Two: RISK FACTORS

Part Three: THE BURDEN

FOREWORDS

A message from

John R Seffrin, PhD
Chief Executive Officer
American Cancer Society

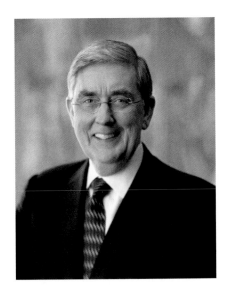

Cancer is potentially one of the most preventable and curable chronic life-threatening diseases. Nevertheless, in 2002 there were an estimated 11 million new cancer cases and nearly 7 million cancer deaths worldwide. By 2020, more than 16 million new cancer cases and 10 million deaths are expected. Seventy percent of these deaths will likely occur in developing countries that are unprepared to address their growing cancer burdens.

We know cancer can be controlled. Declining mortality rates for many cancers in developed nations prove it. But without aggressive intervention, similar results may not be seen elsewhere. Real progress requires a concerted effort at all levels of society. That's why the American Cancer Society and the International Union Against Cancer offer programmes designed to help the global cancer community – especially emerging cancer societies – achieve long-term success in cancer control. Along with our partners at the Centers for Disease Control and Prevention and International Agency for Cancer Research, we are working to lay a foundation for global cancer control and prevention.

Because these organizations share ambitious goals, I am proud to welcome the timely publication of *The Cancer Atlas*, another important step in our collective effort. Here are compelling, evidence-based data to help cancer control experts around the world combat the disease locally, nationally, and globally. Information is a powerful tool in the hands of passionate, dedicated individuals, and this book is an important new resource to arm and inform cancer control professionals worldwide.

In addition to the leading-edge information we need to inform our cancer control strategies, *The Cancer Atlas* also provides an intangible, powerful weapon – hope. The significant and exciting updates chronicled within these pages prove that our broad network of determined cancer control professionals are making a difference for the world. Together, we can empower the developing world to alleviate its cancer burden. With *The Cancer Atlas* in our arsenal, we will continue to move toward victory over cancer.

JOHN R SEFFRIN
Atlanta, USA

A message from

Julie Louise Gerberding, MD, MPH
Director
Centers for Disease Control and Prevention

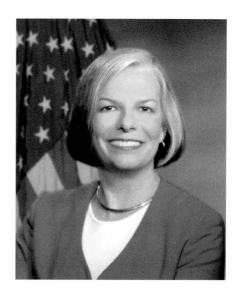

The Centers for Disease Control and Prevention is pleased to have played a role in producing the first-ever *Cancer Atlas*, the third in a series of atlases describing important issues related to chronic diseases worldwide.

The cancer community has made extraordinary progress in many parts of the world. In Europe, death rates for several common cancers are decreasing steadily, and in the USA, death rates from all cancers combined have dropped 1.1 percent per year since 1993. These successes are due in part to public health efforts targeting prevention and early detection of cancer, as well as advances in cancer treatment.

Nonetheless, approximately 11 million people worldwide are diagnosed with cancer annually, and almost 7 million people die of the disease each year. Additionally, more than 25 million people are surviving for years after a cancer diagnosis. A troubling fact is that cancer incidence, survival rates, and quality of life for survivors vary greatly from country to country, depending on differences in exposure to risk factors, availability of public health resources for cancer control efforts, and access to the latest advances in screening and treatment. For example, cervical cancer is the leading cancer in women in developing countries, where organized screening programmes do not exist. In developed countries, where cervical cancer screening is widespread, cervical cancer accounts for only four percent of cancers in women.

To address these disparities, public health agencies and organizations worldwide are assessing local resources, enhancing healthcare infrastructure, and implementing proven cancer-prevention strategies. These strategies must include efforts to prevent the initiation of smoking among adolescents, combat the rise in smoking among women in developing countries, increase the use of proven screening and early-detection methods, and close the large gap in health resources between rich and poor nations.

As the public health community works toward relieving the worldwide burden of cancer, it is important that we consider the entire cancer continuum – from prevention through screening, early detection, diagnosis, treatment, survivorship, palliation, and end-of-life care. To ensure success, we must join forces with researchers, healthcare providers, the private sector, and governments. I encourage you to use this atlas to improve and inform your efforts to prevent and control cancer.

JULIE LOUISE GERBERDING
Atlanta, USA

9

A message from

Peter Boyle
Director of the International Agency for Research on Cancer

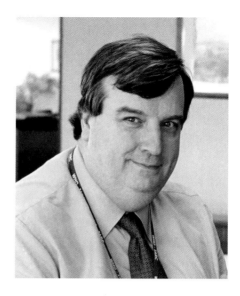

Forty years ago, when the International Agency for Research on Cancer (IARC) was established, cancer was a disease largely confined to the industrialized, high-resource countries. Today, in marked contrast, the majority of the global cancer burden is in low- and medium-resource countries. This atlas illustrates the global scope of the cancer epidemic – highlighting the variations, similarities and sex differences in cancer incidence and deaths. While there are several clearly identified risk factors and we are steadily learning about additional risk factors, there remains a significant proportion of the global cancer burden that we are unable to explain, or advocate steps to avoid, within our current knowledge. The atlas also highlights the importance of cancer surveillance systems, including registries, and of cancer research. These are essential to our understanding of the epidemic, of planning resources, and of taking preventive action.

The IARC is part of the World Health Organization. The Agency's work has four main objectives: monitoring global cancer occurrence, identifying the causes of cancer, elucidating the mechanisms of carcinogenesis, and developing scientific strategies for cancer control. The role of IARC among cancer research institutes is characterized by its focus on research of direct relevance to cancer prevention in international populations, by its emphasis on studies that combine epidemiological and laboratory approaches, and by the special forum and support it provides for international collaborations.

The main emphasis of IARC's research programme is on epidemiology and environmental carcinogenesis and IARC also makes a significant contribution in the area of research training. This emphasis reflects the generally accepted notion that 80 percent of all cancers are, directly or indirectly, linked to environmental factors, and thus are potentially preventable; second, the recent recognition of the fact that epidemiology may play an important part in cancer prevention and in the evaluation of prevention measures; lastly, the fact that geographical variations in cancer incidence almost certainly reflect differences in the environment and are therefore particularly well suited for international research efforts.

Epidemiological research is thus orientated towards two areas: on the one hand, descriptive studies show the trends of cancer incidence and mortality in different populations and geographical areas and, on the other hand, analytical studies focus on the relationships between incidence and mortality and specific risk factors (tobacco use, alcohol consumption, chronic infections, diet, some professional exposures, etc). IARC is, therefore, different from all other research institutes, in that it brings an international dimension to studies on human cancer and the relationships of people and their environment.

I commend the authors of this atlas for bringing a strong sense of the global nature of the cancer burden throughout this book. As Director of the IARC, I am very pleased to see that much of the data used in this atlas is from the IARC database, thus giving the collected statistics a wider audience.

PETER BOYLE
Lyon, France

PREFACE

With full-colour maps and graphics, this atlas illustrates the world's cancer burden and describes efforts to address that burden. It also includes historical highlights, predictions for the future and useful contact information. Readers will learn about the various risk factors for cancer; the costs of cancer; the remarkable differences and similarities in the patterns of cancer around the world; and efforts to prevent, detect and treat cancer. The atlas is for anyone concerned about cancer, including cancer survivors, their families and friends. It is also for those concerned with health policy, public health, health economics, gender issues, resource allocation and human development.

Highlighting the fact that the burden of cancer is increasing in developing countries, which have fewer resources to address the problem, the atlas asserts the importance of a multifaceted approach to reducing the burden of cancer. Such an approach requires the participation of governmental agencies in many nations, the business sector, non-profit organizations, the World Health Organization and the general public. In short, it requires the input of all of civil society.

The anti-cancer movement has developed many successful strategies contributing to the control of cancer around the world, and this atlas highlights a few of those successes, including the establishment of cancer registries; research efforts in developing and developed countries; breakthroughs in prevention, early detection and treatment; and improvements in the lives of those affected by cancer.

JUDITH MACKAY
Asian Consultancy on Tobacco Control
Hong Kong SAR, China

AHMEDIN JEMAL
American Cancer Society
Atlanta, USA

NANCY C LEE
Centers for Disease Control and Prevention
Atlanta, USA

D MAXWELL PARKIN
University of Oxford
UK

ACKNOWLEDGEMENTS

Particular thanks go to the American Cancer Society and to the Centers for Disease Control and Prevention, USA, for their generous financial support of this atlas, and to the International Agency for Research on Cancer for their helpful comments. The International Union Against Cancer (UICC) supplied much helpful information, for which we are grateful. We would also like to thank the World Health Organization, in particular the International Agency for Research on Cancer, for supplying datasets, and for useful suggestions and advice.

Many people have helped in the preparation of this atlas. We would particularly like to thank our principal researchers: Brook Raflo, Division of Cancer Prevention and Control, Centers for Disease Control and Prevention, USA; Nicole Schrag, Department of Epidemiology and Surveillance Research, American Cancer Society, USA.

We would like to acknowledge the following people at the American Cancer Society and the Centers for Disease Control and Prevention: Kevin Brady, Division of Cancer Prevention and Control, Centers for Disease Control and Prevention, USA; Ralph Coates, Division of Cancer Prevention and Control, Centers for Disease Control and Prevention, USA; Michael Thun, Epidemiology and Surveillance Research, American Cancer Society, USA; Elizabeth Ward, Epidemiology and Surveillance Research, American Cancer Society, USA.

For their advice on particular maps and subjects, we would like to thank the following:

1 Mechanism of tumour development
Elsevier Ltd: diagram on page 21 (top) based on diagram from *European Journal of Cancer, Vol 36*: 1589-1594, Wyke JA: Overview: burgeoning promise… © 2000 Elsevier Ltd with permission from Elsevier.

2 Risk factors
Robert C Burton, National Cancer Control Initiative, Australia; Cynthia Jorgensen, Division of Cancer Prevention and Control, Centers for Disease Control and Prevention, USA; Mona Saraiya, Division of Cancer Prevention and Control, Centers for Disease Control and Prevention, USA.

3 Risks for boys and **4 Risks for girls**
Cheryll J Cardinez, Division of Cancer Prevention and Control, Centers for Disease Control and Prevention, USA; Yumiko Mochizuki-Kobayashi, Tobacco Free Initiative, World Health Organization; Wick Warren, Office on Smoking and Health, Centers for Disease Control and Prevention, USA.

5 Tobacco
Jaclynn Lippe, Department of Chronic Diseases and Health Promotion, World Health Organization; Kate Strong, Surveillance and Information for Policy, World Health Organization.

8 Ultraviolet radiation
Bruce Gordon, Richard Mackay, Eva Rehfuess, authors of *Inheriting the World: The Atlas of Children's Health and the Environment* (WHO, 2004) © Myriad Editions/www.MyriadEditions.com for permission to reproduce **The sun's rays** map.

13 Major cancers
Jacques Ferlay, International Agency for Research on Cancer.

14 Cancer in children
Dr Eva Steliarova-Foucher, International Agency for Research on Cancer.

15 Cancer survivors
Darnelle Bernier, International Relay For Life, American Cancer Society, USA; Jose Julio Divino, Campaign and Communications Cluster, International Union Against Cancer; Lori A Pollack, Division of Cancer Prevention and Control, Centers for Disease Control and Prevention, USA.

16 Economic costs
Evan H Blecher, School of Economics, University of Cape Town, South Africa; Corne P van Walbeek, School of Economics, University of Cape Town, South Africa.

18 Cancer registries
The International Association of Cancer Registries.

20 Primary prevention
Andri Aristotelous, Ministry of Health, Cyprus; Immaculada Castro Rodriguez, Dirección General de Salud Pública, Consejería de Sanidad y Consumo, Murcia, Spain; Ian G Catchpole, Ipsos Health, UK; Jacques Fracheboud, Dept of Public Health, Netherlands; Michael Keighley, Chairman, Public Affairs Committee, United European Gastroenterology Federation, UK; Paola Mantellini, Istituto Scientifico della Regione Toscana, Italy; Lola Salas Trejo, Jefa de Unidad de Prevención de Cáncer, Oficina Plan del Cáncer, Dirección General de Salud Pública, Consellería de Sanitat, Valencia, Spain; Maja Primicakelj, Professor, Institute of Oncology, Slovenia; Raquel Zubizarreta Alberdi, Jefa de Servicio, Dirección Xeral de Saúde Pública, Consellería de Sanidade, Galicia, Spain.

24 Cancer organizations
Brita Baker, International Union Against Cancer; Italo Goyzueta, International Union Against Cancer; Luis Guillermo, La Sociedad Anticancerosa de Venezuela; Ruben Israel, GLOBALink Information Services, International Union Against Cancer; Nancy E Lins, American Cancer Society, USA; Isabel Mortara, International Union Against Cancer.

25 Health education
Marjo Pyykönen, International Quit&Win, Finland; Geoff Thaxter and Marianne C Naafs-Wilstra, International Confederation of Childhood Cancer Parent Organizations.

26 Policies and legislation
Douglas Bettcher, WHO Framework Convention on Tobacco Control Office, Tobacco Free Initiative, World Health Organization.

27 The future
George TJ Au, Clinical oncologist, Hong Kong; Neville Rigby and Rachel Jackson Leach, International Association for the Study of Obesity/International Obesity Task Force.

The history of cancer
George TJ Au, Clinical oncologist, Hong Kong; Brigitta Blaha-Silva, Consul-General, Hong Kong; Chris Carrigan, National Cancer Registry Coordinator, UK.

For their diverse talents and editorial expertise, and individual as well as collective contributions, we would like to thank the team at Myriad Editions: Candida Lacey, Corinne Pearlman, Isabelle Lewis, Jannet King and Sadie Mayne.

Finally, we want to thank our respective families for their support during the preparation of this atlas.

PHOTO CREDITS

The publishers are grateful to the following organizations and photographers for permission to reproduce their photographs:

Front cover
Girl using sun protection © Colin Kennedy

Back cover (left to right)
Test tubes © American Cancer Society Inc/John Tarantino 2005
Youth smoking, Bangladesh. WHO-393048 © WHO/Harry Anenden
Survivor handprints at Relay for Life event © American Cancer Society Inc/Rick Nahmias 2005
Lungs © American Cancer Society Inc 2005
Cancer survivors lap at Relay event © American Cancer Society Inc/Rick Nahmias 2005

Part One: Introduction
Survivor handprints at Relay for Life event © American Cancer Society/Rick Nahmias 2005

Part Two: Risk Factors
Youth smoking, Bangladesh. WHO-393048 © WHO/Harry Anenden

Part Three: The Burden
Doctor pointing to chest x-ray © American Cancer Society Inc 2005

Part Four: Economics
Stethoscope over dollar bills. istock 837203 © Andrej Tchernov

Part Five: Taking Action
Cancer survivors lap at Relay event © American Cancer Society Inc/Rick Nahmias 2005

Part Six: The Future & the Past
Hands © American Cancer Society Inc/Nelda Mays 2004

Part Seven: World Tables
Fruit and vegetables © American Cancer Society Inc 2004

1 Mechanism of tumour development
Two women talking. NM0207/3698. © American Cancer Society Inc/Nelda Mays 2005

7 Diet and nutrition
Fruit and vegetables ©American Cancer Society Inc 2004

Meat consumption © The World Bank/Alejandro Lipszyc

8 Ultraviolet radiation
Girl in pink top © American Cancer Society Inc/Chris Hamilton 2005
Woman and child © American Cancer Society Inc/Richard Gaskins 2001

9 Reproductive and hormonal factors
Woman and baby © UNICEF India/Amar Talwar 1986

10 The risk of getting cancer
Man and woman © American Cancer Society Inc/Chris Hamilton 2005

13 Lung cancer
Lungs © American Cancer Society Inc 2005

14 Cancer in children
Pie charts:
USA (black), Europe (white), Latin America © American Cancer Society Inc/Chris Hamilton 2005;
East Asia © American Cancer Society Inc/ John Tarantino 2004; Africa © Ami Vitale/ World Bank; India ©UNICEF India/ Ami Vitale Boy and girl blowing bubbles ©American Cancer Society Inc 2005

15 Cancer survivors
Relay for Life © American Cancer Society Inc 2004

19 Research
Test tubes © American Cancer Society Inc/John Tarantino 2005

21 Prevention: population and systems approaches
Shade structure © Nancy Lee 2000

24 Cancer organizations
Poster © The Venezuela Cancer Society (VCS)/ Sociedad Anticancerosa de Venezuela (SAV)

25 Health education
Thailand World Cancer Day 2003 © WHO/H Anenden

27 The future
Amy, Hong Kong © Guy Nowell

14

ABOUT THE AUTHORS

Dr Judith Mackay is a medical doctor based in Hong Kong. She is a Senior Policy Advisor to the World Health Organization, and holds professorships at the Chinese Academy of Preventive Medicine in Beijing, and the Department of Community Medicine at the University of Hong Kong. After an early career as a hospital physician, she moved to working in preventive and public health. She is a Fellow of the Royal Colleges of Physicians of Edinburgh and of London. Dr Mackay has received many international awards, including the WHO Commemorative Medal, a Royal Award from the King of Thailand, the Fries Prize for Improving Health, the Luther Terry Award for Outstanding Individual Leadership, the International Partnering for World Health Award, and the Founding International Achievement Award from the Asia Pacific Association for the Control of Tobacco. She co-authored the first and second edition of *The Tobacco Atlas* and is the author of several other Myriad atlases, including *The State of Health Atlas*, *The Penguin Atlas of Human Sexual Behavior* and *The Atlas of Heart Disease and Stroke*.

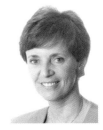

Dr Ahmedin Jemal is Program Director of Cancer Occurrence at the American Cancer Society based in Atlanta. He currently holds an adjunct faculty position at the Rollins School of Public Health of Emory University, USA. His main research interests include cancer surveillance and stimulating the application of existing cancer control knowledge into practice. He is the author and co-author of many scientific articles in peer-reviewed journals.

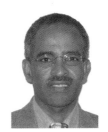

Dr Nancy C Lee works as a consultant for the US Centers for Disease Control and Prevention (CDC) in the areas of public health, epidemiology, and cancer control. She has 24 years of experience with the CDC, and from 1999-2004 served as Director of CDC's Division of Cancer Prevention and Control. Her efforts there focused on cancer surveillance, prevention, screening and early detection, and development of the USA's public health efforts in cancer control.

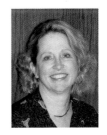

Dr D Maxwell Parkin is an epidemiologist attached to the Clinical Trials Service Unit and Epidemiological Studies Unit at the University of Oxford, UK. He worked at the International Agency for Research on Cancer from 1981-2004 as head of the Descriptive Epidemiology Unit. He is currently President of the International Association of Cancer Registries (IACR). His main research interests are in descriptive epidemiology (international cancer patterns and trends), with a major concern for cancer registration, and in early detection (screening) for cancer. He has published more than 300 papers in the international scientific literature.

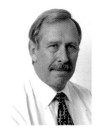

GLOSSARY

Adenocarcinoma – cancer that begins in cells that line certain internal organs and that have glandular properties (the ability to generate a substance).

Aflatoxin – harmful substance made by certain types of Aspergillus mould that may be found on poorly stored grains and nuts. Consumption of foods contaminated with aflatoxin is a risk factor for hepatocellular (liver) cancer.

Age-specific rate – a rate for a specified age group. The numerator and denominator refer to the same age group.

Age standardization – a technique that allows comparison of incidence (or mortality) rates between populations, without the effect of any differences that are due to their age structures. The Age-Standardized Rate (ASR) used in this atlas is the rate that a population would have if it had the same age structure as a "standard" population. The most frequently used standard population is the world standard population. The calculated incidence or mortality rate is then called the world age standardized incidence or mortality rate. It is expressed as a rate per 100,000.

Asbestos – a natural material that is made of tiny fibres and used in insulation. Asbestos exposure is a risk factor for several cancers, including lung cancer.

Benign tumour – an abnormal growth that is not cancer and does not spread to other areas of the body.

Body mass index (BMI) – a measure of a person's weight in relation to his or her height calculated as weight in kilogrammes divided by height in metres squared.

Cancer – a disease in which abnormal cells divide uncontrollably. Cancer cells can invade nearby tissues, and spread through the bloodstream and lymphatic system to other parts of the body.

Cancer screening programmes – programmes organized at a national or regional level that have (1) an explicit policy, (2) a team responsible for organizing the screening and delivering appropriate healthcare, and (3) a structure for assuring quality screening and follow-up of abnormal screening tests.
- national screening programme: population-based screening programme organized at the national level
- sub-national screening programme: population-based screening programme organized at the sub-national level
- pilot screening programme: pilot population-based screening programme, typically organized at the sub-national level
- public health policy only: established national policy for cancer screening, but no population-based screening programme (in the USA, opportunistic screening and organized programmes for HMO private health provider members and low-income qualified individuals are available).

Carcinogen – any substance – chemical, physical or biologic – that causes cancer. Examples include tobacco smoke, asbestos, human papillomavirus and ultraviolet radiation.

Carcinoma – a cancerous tumour that begins in the lining layer (epithelial cells) of organs. At least 80% of all cancers are carcinomas.

Cervical cancer – cancer of the lower, narrow end of the uterus that forms a canal between the uterus and vagina. Development of cervical cancer requires previous infection with human papillomavirus (HPV).

Chemotherapy – treatment with drugs to destroy cancer cells. Chemotherapy may be used alone, or in combination with surgery or radiation, to treat cancer when the cancer has spread, when the cancer has come back (recurred), or when there is a strong chance that the cancer could recur.

Cobalt machines – use a radioactive form of the metal cobalt as a source of radiation to treat cancer.

Colonoscopy – examination of the colon with a long, flexible, lighted tube called a colonoscope. The doctor looks for polyps or early cancers during the exam and removes them using a wire passed through the colonoscope.

Computerized Tomography (CT) – a series of detailed pictures of areas inside the body taken from different angles; the pictures are created by a computer linked to an x-ray machine. Also called computerized axial tomography (CAT) scan. A special kind of CT machine, the spiral CT, has been used to look for early lung cancer, but it is still uncertain whether such a test will be an effective cancer screening tool.

Developed countries – the United Nations Population Division divides the world's regions into two categories – "more developed" and "less developed." The more developed regions include Australia/New Zealand, Europe, Northern America, and Japan.

Developing countries – the United Nations Population Division divides the world's regions into two categories – "more developed" and "less developed." The less developed regions which this atlas calls "developing countries" include all the regions of Africa, Asia (excluding Japan), Latin America, and the Caribbean, as well as Melanesia, Micronesia, and Polynesia. The World Bank excludes from "developing" regions such affluent countries as Singapore.

Diagnosis – the process of identifying a disease by the signs and symptoms, as well as medical tests and tissue biopsy as needed.

Direct costs – expenditures for medical procedures and services associated with the treatment and care of people with cancer.

Electron accelerator machines – used in medical radiation therapy, these machines accelerate tiny charged particles called electrons, and deliver uniform doses of high-energy x-ray to the region of the patient's tumour. These x-rays can destroy the cancer cells while sparing the surrounding normal tissue.

Endometrial cancer – cancer of the layer of tissue that lines the uterus. A risk factor for endometrial cancer is exposure to excess amounts of the hormone oestrogen.

Exogenous hormones – hormones that are derived from outside the body, such as oral contraceptives and hormone replacement therapy.

Epidemic – occurrence of an illness, condition or behaviour that affects many people in the same region during a specified period of time. To constitute an epidemic, this occurrence must exceed normal occurrence in the region.

European Union 25 (EU-25) – Austria, Belgium, Cyprus, Czech Republic, Denmark, Estonia, Finland, France, Germany, Greece, Hungary, Ireland, Italy, Latvia, Lithuania, Luxembourg, Malta, the Netherlands, Poland, Portugal, Slovak Republic (Slovakia), Slovenia, Spain, Sweden and UK.

Faecal occult blood test – a test used to screen for colorectal cancer. It looks for hidden blood in the stools, the presence of which could be a sign of cancer.

Hepatocellular carcinoma – the most common type of cancer originating in the liver.

Hormone replacement therapy (HRT) – hormones (oestrogen, progesterone, or other types) given to women after menopause to replace the hormones no longer produced by the ovaries.

Human papillomavirus (HPV) – a virus that can cause abnormal tissue growth and other changes to cells. Infection with certain types of HPV increases the risk of developing cervical cancer.

Incidence – the number of new cases of cancer that occur in a defined population during a specified period of time. "Incidence rate" is the rate at which new cases occur in a population, and is calculated by dividing the number of new cases that occur during a specified time period by the total number of people in the defined population.

Indirect costs – costs related to – but not immediately associated with – the detection, diagnosis and treatment of cancer. These may include lost income due to premature death, short-term or long-term disability, and psychological costs.

Kaposi sarcoma – a type of cancer characterized by the abnormal growth of blood vessels that develop into skin lesions or occur internally. It is caused by Human herpesvirus-8. The risk of developing Kaposi sarcoma in a person who has Human herpesvirus-8 increases significantly if the person also has the virus that causes AIDS.

Leukaemia – cancer of the blood or blood-forming organs.

Lumpectomy – surgery to remove a breast lump or tumour and a small amount of surrounding normal tissue.

Lymphoma – a cancer of the lymphatic system. The lymphatic system is a network of thin vessels and nodes throughout the body. The two main types of lymphoma are Hodgkin lymphoma (or disease) and non-Hodgkin lymphoma. The treatment methods for these two types of lymphomas are different.

Malignant tumour – a mass of cancer cells that may invade surrounding tissues or spread (metastasize) to distant areas of the body.

Melanoma – a cancerous (malignant) tumour that begins in the cells that produce the skin coloring (melanocytes). Melanoma is almost always curable in its early stages. However, it is likely to spread, and once it has spread to other parts of the body the chances for a cure decrease.

Menarche – the first menstrual period, usually occurring during puberty.

Menopause – the time period marked by the permanent cessation of menstruation, usually occurring between the ages of 45 and 55.

Metastasis – the distant spread of cancer from its primary site to other parts of the body.

Morbidity – any departure from physiological or psychological well-being. Measures of morbidity for people living with cancer may include disability, pain, time away from work, or days spent in the hospital.

Mortality – the number of deaths from cancer that occur in a population during a specified period of time. Mortality rate is the rate at which deaths occur in a population, and is calculated by dividing the number of deaths that occur during a specified period of time by the number of people in the specified population.

Ovarian cancer – cancer occurring in one of a pair of female reproductive glands in which the ova, or eggs, are formed. The ovaries are located in the pelvis, one on each side of the uterus.

Neoplasm – an abnormal growth (tumour) that starts from a single altered cell; a neoplasm may be benign or malignant. Cancer is a malignant neoplasm.

Neuroblastoma – cancer that arises in immature nerve cells and affects mostly infants and children.

Palliative care – an approach that aims to improve the quality of life for patients and families facing the problems associated with life-threatening cancers. It provides for prevention and relief of suffering, through treatment for pain and other symptoms, as well as through spiritual and psychosocial support, at the time of cancer diagnosis, through the end of life, and during family bereavement.

Prevalence – a measure of the proportion of persons in the population with a certain disease, condition or behaviour at a given time.

Prognosis – prediction of the course of a cancer, and the outlook for a cure.

Radiotherapy – the use of radiation to kill cancer cells or stop them from dividing.

Radon – a radioactive gas that is released by uranium, a substance found in soil and rock. Radon is a risk factor for lung cancer.

Retinoblastoma – a rare form of eye cancer that affects the retina of infants and young children.

Sarcoma – a cancer of the bone, cartilage, fat, muscle, blood vessels, or other connective or supportive tissue.

Sigmoidoscopy – a test to help find cancer or polyps on the inside of the rectum and part of the colon. A slender, hollow, lighted tube is placed into the rectum. The doctor is able to look for polyps or other abnormalities. The sigmoidoscope is shorter than the colonoscope.

Solar irradiation – see ultraviolet radiation below.

Survival – the proportion (or percentage) of persons with a given cancer who are still alive after a specified time period (eg 1, 3, or 5 years) following diagnosis.

Total fertility rate – average number of births during a woman's lifetime, given current childbearing patterns.

Ultraviolet (UV) radiation – invisible rays that are part of the energy that comes from the sun. UV radiation also comes from sun lamps and tanning beds. UV radiation can damage the skin, lead to premature aging, and cause melanoma and other types of skin cancer.

Wilms tumour – a type of kidney cancer that usually occurs in children younger than 5 years of age.

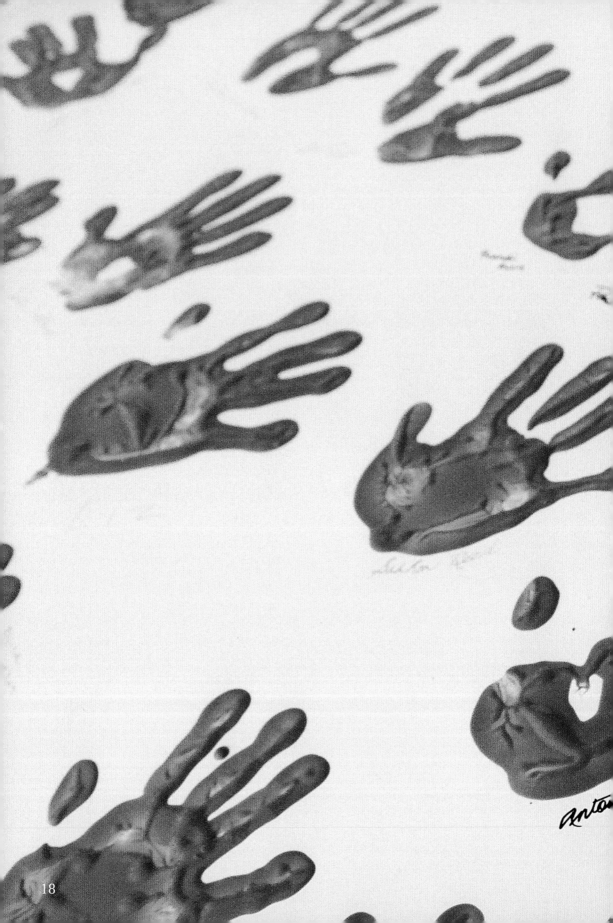

PART ONE

INTRODUCTION

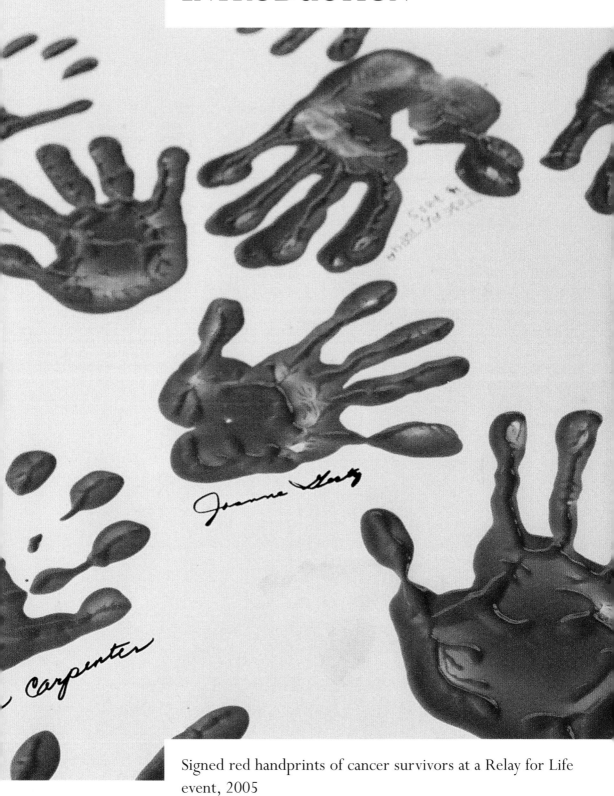

Signed red handprints of cancer survivors at a Relay for Life event, 2005

1 | Mechanism of tumour development

"We are all cells in the same body of humanity."
Peace Pilgrim,
born Mildred Lisette Norman Ryder,
writer and activist (1908–81)

Normal cells divide, mature and die. Cancer develops when abnormal cells in the body do not follow this progression.

Cancer begins with damage to one or more genes in a single cell. This damage can cause the cell to divide incorrectly and to produce abnormal cells. If the body's immune system does not repair or destroy these abnormal cells, then the newer cells can become even more abnormal, eventually producing cancer cells. Cancer cells also divide more rapidly than do normal cells, and usually do not function normally. Eventually, cancer cells may begin to pile on top of nearby cells, forming a mass of tissue called a tumour. The process by which a normal cell becomes a cancerous tumour usually takes years.

The term "stage" describes the extent or severity of a person's cancer. During early stages of cancer, a person may have only one small, cancerous tumour. More advanced stages may involve a larger tumour, the spread of cancer to lymph nodes, or the spread of cancer to other parts of the body (metastases).

To determine the likelihood that a person will recover from cancer (prognosis), physicians look at many factors, including the type and stage of cancer.

Not all cancers form solid tumours. Leukaemia cancer cells are found in blood and blood-forming organs.

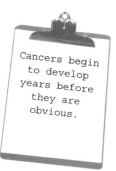

Cancers begin to develop years before they are obvious.

STAGE OF CANCER

precancerous abnormal cells | localized cancer | regional cancer | metastatic cancer

PROGNOSIS

better

worse

Stage and prognosis
The prognosis, or likelihood that a person will recover from cancer, is related to the type and stage of cancer. Generally, the prognosis is better during earlier stages.

Cancers
that develop slowly
may present opportunities
for early detection.

How a tumour develops

Damage to genes in a single cell (mutations) can lead to progressively more abnormal cells. Eventually, abnormal cells may become cancerous cells, which often divide quickly and do not die.

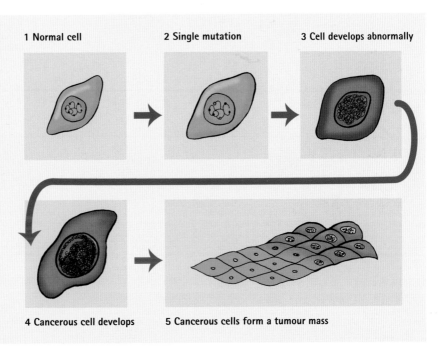

1 Normal cell

2 Single mutation

3 Cell develops abnormally

4 Cancerous cell develops

5 Cancerous cells form a tumour mass

How a tumour spreads

Metastases happen when cancer cells from the original tumour spread to different parts of the body, and eventually form secondary tumours at sites distant from the original tumour.

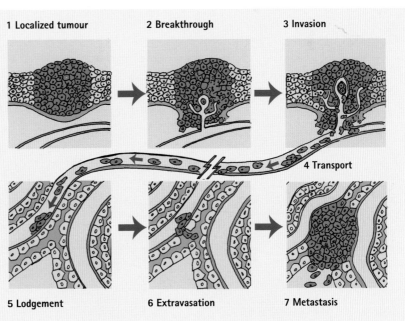

1 Localized tumour

2 Breakthrough

3 Invasion

4 Transport

5 Lodgement

6 Extravasation

7 Metastasis

21

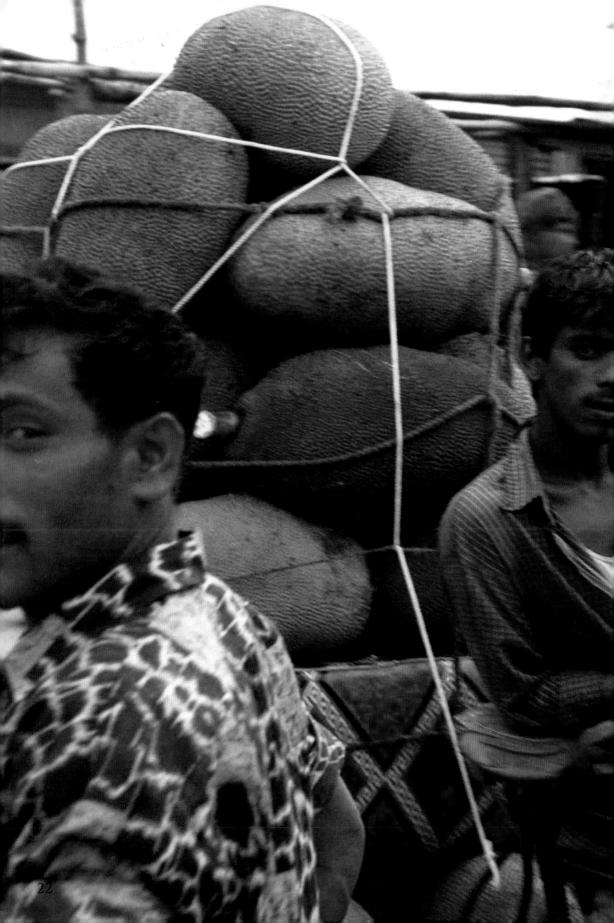

RISK FACTORS

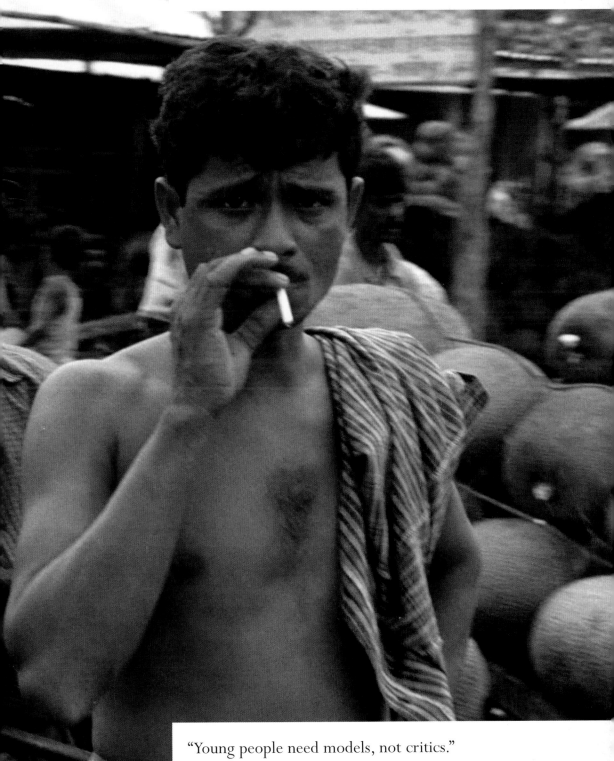

"Young people need models, not critics."

John Wooden, American basketball coach

Risk factors

Many factors contribute to the changes in a cell that result in cancer. These risk factors may be intrinsic to an individual, such as sex, age, or genes. But most are external, in the individual's general environment. The interplay between the intrinsic and external factors is the major determinant of an individual's cancer risk.

Risk factors vary widely worldwide based on differences in lifestyle and in social, economic and political development. Topography, climate and other environmental characteristics play a less important role in the variability of risk factors.

Fortunately, cancer researchers have identified many factors that may be modified to reduce cancer risk. Some require individual behaviour change; others require changes at the population level, by employers or communities, for example. Improvement in these risk factors is most effectively addressed by both. For example, a mother needs to take her infant for hepatitis B immunization; her government must ensure the immunization is accessible and affordable.

The most important modifiable risk factors for cancer are tobacco use, a diet high in saturated fats and with an insufficient intake of fresh fruits and vegetables, and infection with viruses or bacteria that cause cancer.

Proportion of cancers caused by major risk factors

In developing countries, chronic infections are a major cause of cancer and occupational carcinogens pose a substantial risk.

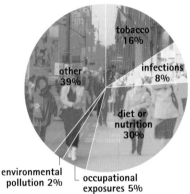

developed countries

tobacco 16%
infections 8%
diet or nutrition 30%
other 39%
environmental pollution 2%
occupational exposures 5%

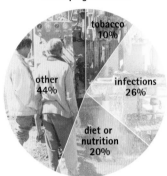

developing countries

tobacco 10%
infections 26%
diet or nutrition 20%
other 44%

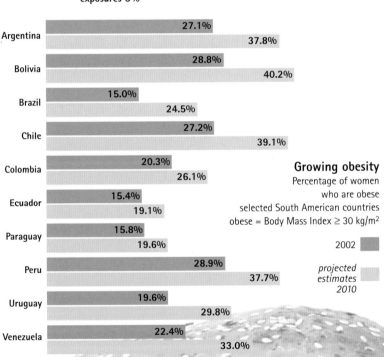

	2002	projected estimates 2010
Argentina	27.1%	37.8%
Bolivia	28.8%	40.2%
Brazil	15.0%	24.5%
Chile	27.2%	39.1%
Colombia	20.3%	26.1%
Ecuador	15.4%	19.1%
Paraguay	15.8%	19.6%
Peru	28.9%	37.7%
Uruguay	19.6%	29.8%
Venezuela	22.4%	33.0%

Growing obesity
Percentage of women who are obese selected South American countries
obese = Body Mass Index ≥ 30 kg/m^2

2002
projected estimates 2010

Obesity and income
Percentage classified as obese in each household-income quintile
2002–03

Canada
USA

	1st (poorest)	2nd	3rd	4th	5th (richest)
Canada	17.6%	16.6%	16.2%	14.4%	12.7%
USA	27.3%	23.4%	19.4%	19.5%	14.8%

Major modifiable risk factors

- **Tobacco use**
  Tobacco use is the main cause of cancers of the lung, larynx, oral cavity, and oesophagus, and a major cause of bladder and pancreas cancers.

- **Unhealthy diet**
  Up to 30% of cancers in developed countries may be related to poor nutrition. Diets high in saturated fats and low in fruits and vegetables increase the risk of cancers of the breast, colon, prostate and oesophagus.

- **Infectious agents**
  Infectious agents account for 18% of cancers worldwide. Human papillomavirus, hepatitis B virus, and the *Helicobacter pylori* bacterium account for the largest number of cancers due to infections.

- **Ultraviolet radiation**
  Sunlight is the major source of UV radiation, which causes several types of skin cancer, the most common malignancy in humans.

- **Physical inactivity**
  A sedentary lifestyle increases the risk of colon cancer, and may increase the risk for other types of cancer. Its effects are closely related to an individual's nutrition.

> Many cancer risk factors can be changed for the better.

Other modifiable risk factors

- **Alcohol use**
  Heavy alcohol use causes cancers of the oral cavity, oesophagus, liver and upper respiratory tract. The cancer risk is greatly increased by concurrent smoking. Alcohol use also increases the risk of breast cancer.

- **Occupational exposures**
  Certain substances encountered at work are carcinogens, including asbestos, arsenic, benzene, silica and second-hand tobacco smoke. Lung cancer is the most common occupational cancer.

- **Socioeconomic status**
  Some cancers occur more often in people with a higher socioeconomic status (SES); others are more common in lower-SES populations. SES is most likely a marker for lifestyle and other risk factors described in this section.

- **Environmental pollution**
  Pollution of air, water and soil account for between 1% and 4% of all cancers in developed nations.

- **Obesity**
  Obesity is an important risk factor for endometrial, kidney, gallbladder and breast cancers.

- **Food contaminants**
  Certain food contaminants are carcinogenic, including those that occur naturally (eg aflatoxins) and those that are manufactured (eg pesticides).

- **Ionizing radiation**
  For most, the greatest exposure to ionizing radiation comes from medical X-rays. But we are all exposed to small amounts of naturally occurring radiation.

Non-modifiable risk factors

- **Ageing**
  The risk of most types of cancer increases with age. The highest cancer rates occur among the elderly.

- **Ethnicity or race**
  The risk of many types of cancer varies between racial and ethnic populations. Some of these differences are attributable to genetic differences, but most are due to differences in lifestyle and exposures to cancer-causing agents.

- **Heredity**
  Inherited "cancer" genes may cause 4% of all cancers. Other genes affect our susceptibility to cancer risk factors.

- **Sex**
  Certain cancers occur in only one sex due to different anatomy, eg prostate, uterus. Others occur in both sexes, but at markedly different rates, eg bladder, breast.

Other risk factors

- **Reproductive factors**
  Female hormones, menstrual history, and childbearing affect the risks of breast, endometrial and ovarian cancers.

- **Immunosuppression**
  Certain viruses that suppress the immune system increase the risk of lymphoma and Kaposi sarcoma.

- **Medicinal drugs**
  Some hormonal drugs can cause cancers, while others reduce the risk. Rarely, anti-cancer drugs have caused another cancer years later.

Risks for boys

Generally, risk factors for childhood cancers cannot be reduced by behaviour change. However, certain behaviours that begin at a young age will increase the risk of cancer later in life. The most notable is tobacco use, the leading cause of cancer mortality worldwide. Exposure to infectious diseases, obesity and excessive sunshine, leading a sedentary lifestyle or eating insufficient fruit and vegetables also increase the risk for developing cancer as an adult.

Most tobacco use begins in early adolescence; worldwide, teenage boys are more likely to start smoking than teenage girls. Cancer deaths would be greatly reduced worldwide if the rates at which young people started smoking decreased. Taxation of tobacco products is the most effective strategy to discourage smoking: as prices increase, tobacco use decreases, especially among young smokers. Other important deterrents include bans on all tobacco advertising and promotion, and smoking restrictions as part of a comprehensive campaign.

Up to 30 percent of cancers are related to diet and nutrition. Because young people who develop healthy eating habits early in life are more likely to continue those healthy habits as adults, efforts to assure a healthy diet for children and young people should be part of a comprehensive cancer control strategy.

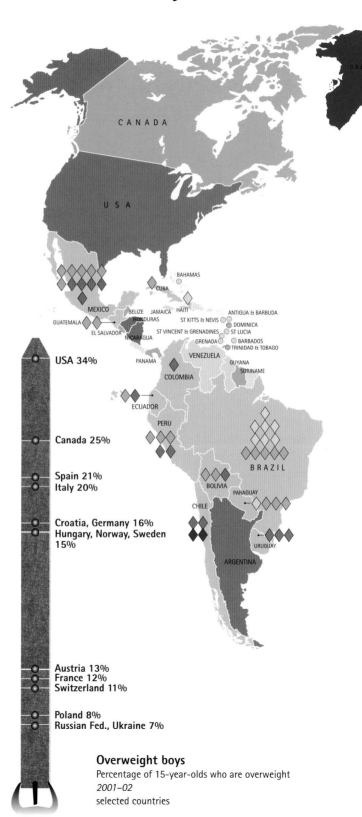

USA 34%

Canada 25%

Spain 21%
Italy 20%

Croatia, Germany 16%
Hungary, Norway, Sweden 15%

Austria 13%
France 12%
Switzerland 11%

Poland 8%
Russian Fed., Ukraine 7%

Overweight boys
Percentage of 15-year-olds who are overweight
2001–02
selected countries

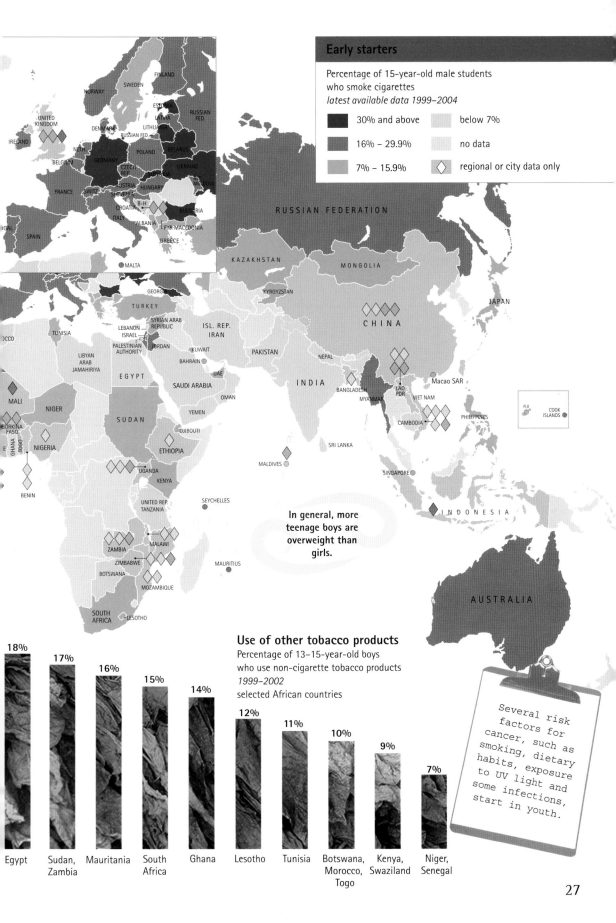

Early starters

Percentage of 15-year-old male students who smoke cigarettes
latest available data 1999–2004

- 30% and above
- 16% – 29.9%
- 7% – 15.9%
- below 7%
- no data
- regional or city data only

In general, more teenage boys are overweight than girls.

Use of other tobacco products

Percentage of 13–15-year-old boys who use non-cigarette tobacco products
1999–2002
selected African countries

Country	%
Egypt	18%
Sudan, Zambia	17%
Mauritania	16%
South Africa	15%
Ghana	14%
Lesotho	12%
Tunisia	11%
Botswana, Morocco, Togo	10%
Kenya, Swaziland	9%
Niger, Senegal	7%

Several risk factors for cancer, such as smoking, dietary habits, exposure to UV light and some infections, start in youth.

Risks for girls

"Children are natural mimics who act like their parents despite every effort to teach them good manners."
Anonymous

Worldwide, tobacco use among adolescents is increasing, especially in developing countries and among girls. In much of Europe and in parts of South America, teenage girls are smoking more than teenage boys.

Obesity is a risk factor for several cancers and increases the risk of dying from many cancers. The most important long-term consequence of childhood obesity is persistence into adulthood.

A lifetime risk of skin cancer is strongly influenced by exposure to the sun during childhood and adolescence, making adequate solar protection more important in childhood than at any other time of life. Lifelong habits to prevent skin cancer should begin during childhood. Effective programmes to promote sun safety in schools exist in some parts of the world, but adolescents are less likely to protect their skin so innovative strategies proven to reduce UV exposure are needed.

An estimated 60 percent of cases of liver cancer worldwide are caused by persistent infections with the hepatitis B virus (HBV). Childhood vaccination programmes against HBV will prevent 90 to 95 percent of these infections and have already been shown to reduce the risk of liver cancer in high-incidence areas.

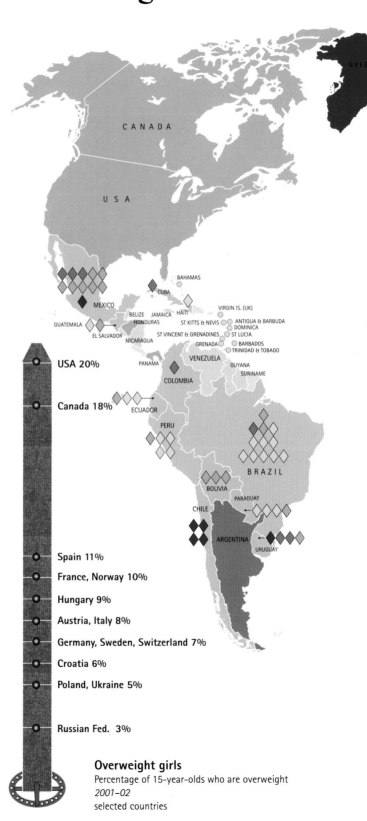

USA 20%

Canada 18%

Spain 11%

France, Norway 10%

Hungary 9%

Austria, Italy 8%

Germany, Sweden, Switzerland 7%

Croatia 6%

Poland, Ukraine 5%

Russian Fed. 3%

Overweight girls
Percentage of 15-year-olds who are overweight
2001–02
selected countries

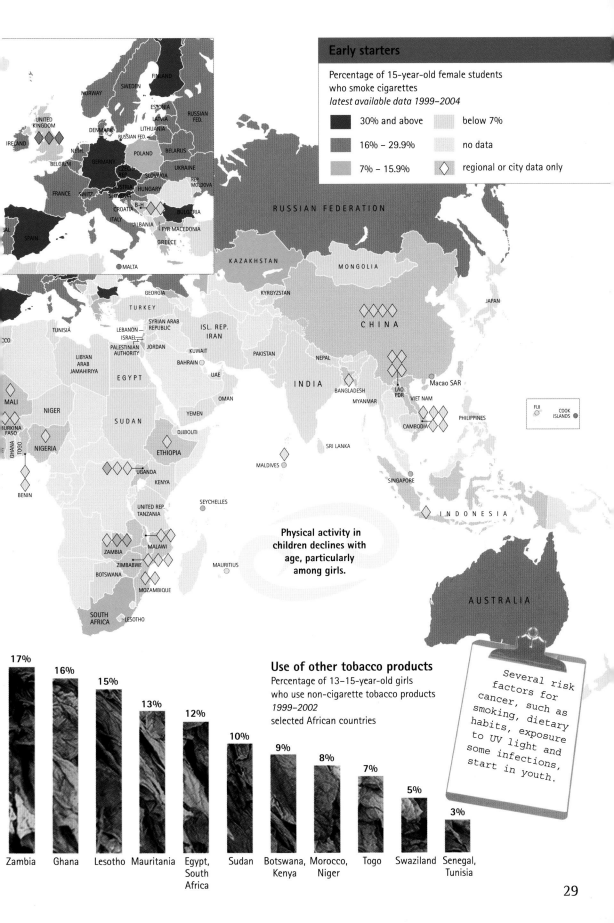

Early starters

Percentage of 15-year-old female students who smoke cigarettes
latest available data 1999–2004

- 30% and above
- 16% – 29.9%
- 7% – 15.9%
- below 7%
- no data
- ◇ regional or city data only

> Physical activity in children declines with age, particularly among girls.

Use of other tobacco products

Percentage of 13–15-year-old girls who use non-cigarette tobacco products
1999–2002
selected African countries

- 17% Zambia
- 16% Ghana
- 15% Lesotho
- 13% Mauritania
- 12% Egypt, South Africa
- 10% Sudan
- 9% Botswana, Kenya
- 8% Morocco, Niger
- 7% Togo
- 5% Swaziland
- 3% Senegal, Tunisia

> Several risk factors for cancer, such as smoking, dietary habits, exposure to UV light and some infections, start in youth.

29

Tobacco

About 1 in 5 cancer deaths worldwide is caused by tobacco.

Globally, the leading causes of death from smoking are: cardiovascular diseases with 1.69 million deaths, cancer with 1.4 million deaths, and chronic obstructive pulmonary disease (COPD) with 0.97 million deaths.

Tobacco is packed with harmful, addictive substances. Scientific evidence has shown conclusively that all forms of tobacco cause cancers (and other diseases). For example, chewing tobacco causes cancer of the lip, tongue and mouth.

Smokers have markedly increased risks of many different cancers. Best known is lung cancer, where tobacco causes 80 percent of lung cancer in men and half of lung cancer in women worldwide. Lung cancer is therefore an almost totally avoidable disease.

In the future, as research proceeds, tobacco may be linked with other cancers.

Exposure to environmental tobacco smoke causes lung and possibly other cancers, as well as other illnesses in non-smoking adults and children.

Lung and other cancers caused by tobacco are often untreatable at the time of diagnosis. The key to reducing these cancers is to prevent initiation of smoking in young people, and to encourage smokers to quit. Quitting smoking substantially reduces cancer risk.

Cancer deaths caused by smoking

Percentage by site of cancer
2005 or most recent estimate

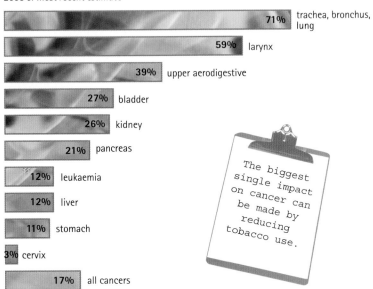

- 71% trachea, bronchus, lung
- 59% larynx
- 39% upper aerodigestive
- 27% bladder
- 26% kidney
- 21% pancreas
- 12% leukaemia
- 12% liver
- 11% stomach
- 3% cervix
- 17% all cancers

The biggest single impact on cancer can be made by reducing tobacco use.

Cancer and tobacco

Cancers caused by tobacco compared with all new cases
2002
millions

Total new cases

- developing countries
- industrialized countries
- attributable to tobacco

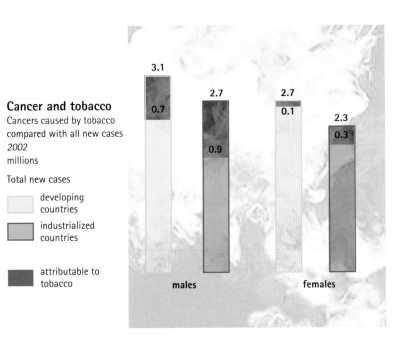

males: 3.1 / 0.7 ... 2.7 / 0.9
females: 2.7 / 0.1 ... 2.3 / 0.3

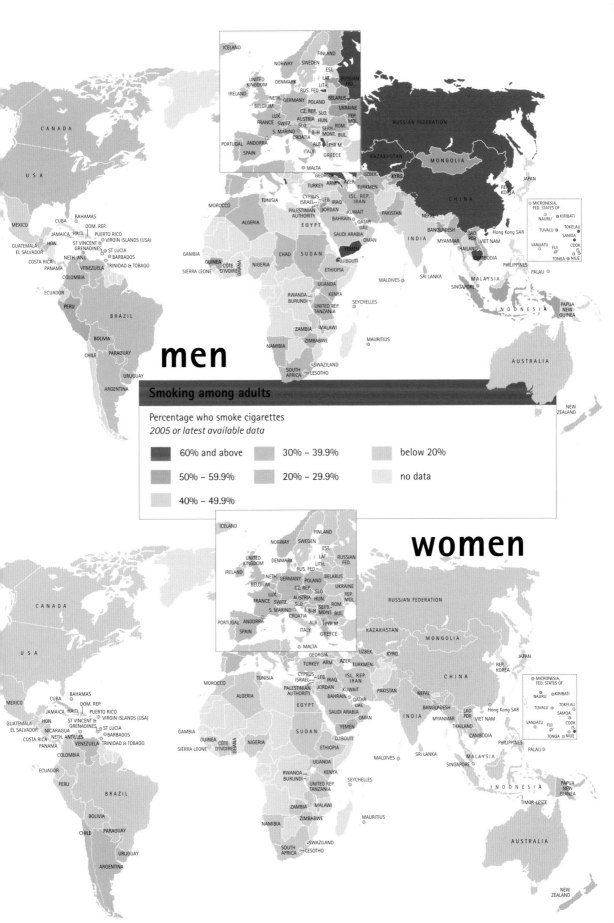

men

women

Smoking among adults

Percentage who smoke cigarettes
2005 or latest available data

- 60% and above
- 50% – 59.9%
- 40% – 49.9%
- 30% – 39.9%
- 20% – 29.9%
- below 20%
- no data

Infection

Infections cause some 1.9 million cases of cancer – 17.8 percent of the global total. The most important agent is the bacterium *Helicobacter pylori* (the cause of 5.6 percent of all cancers), which increases the risk of stomach cancer between five and six fold. Infection with this bacterium is extremely common, especially in developing countries, but is reducing in recent generations.

All cervical cancers result from infection with some 20 types of Human papillomavirus (HPV), as do most of the much rarer cancers of the anus, and probably about half of the cancers of the external genitalia. HPV causes smaller proportions of cancers of the mouth and oro-pharynx, and possibly respiratory cancers.

Chronic infection by the two hepatitis viruses, B (HBV) and C (HCV), is common. Each increases the risk of liver cancer 20 fold or more; together they are responsible for more than 85 percent of the liver cancer in the world. The Epstein-Barr virus, and Human Immunodeficiency Virus (HIV), together with the Human herpesvirus-8, are each responsible for about 100,000 new cancer cases a year. Relatively less important causes of cancer are the schistosomes, Human T-cell Lymphotropic Virus type I, and the liver flukes.

There would be 26.2% fewer cancers in developing countries (1.5 million cases per year) and 7.7% in developed countries (380,000 cases) if these infectious agents were prevented.

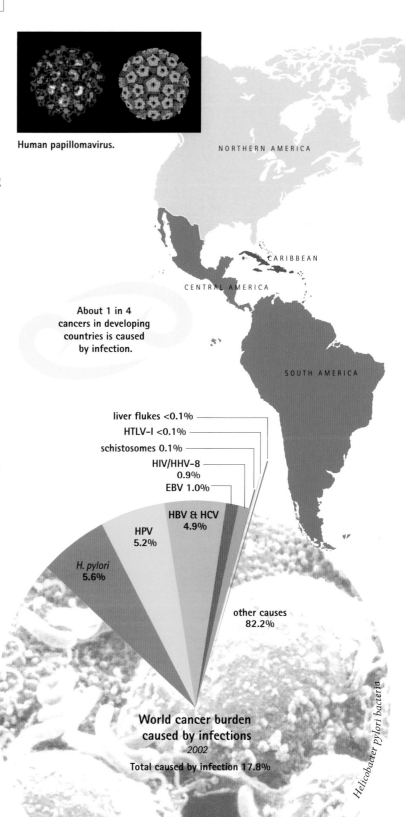

Human papillomavirus.

NORTHERN AMERICA

CARIBBEAN

CENTRAL AMERICA

SOUTH AMERICA

About 1 in 4 cancers in developing countries is caused by infection.

liver flukes <0.1%
HTLV-I <0.1%
schistosomes 0.1%
HIV/HHV-8 0.9%
EBV 1.0%
HBV & HCV 4.9%
HPV 5.2%
H. pylori 5.6%
other causes 82.2%

World cancer burden caused by infections
2002
Total caused by infection 17.8%

Helicobacter pylori bacteria

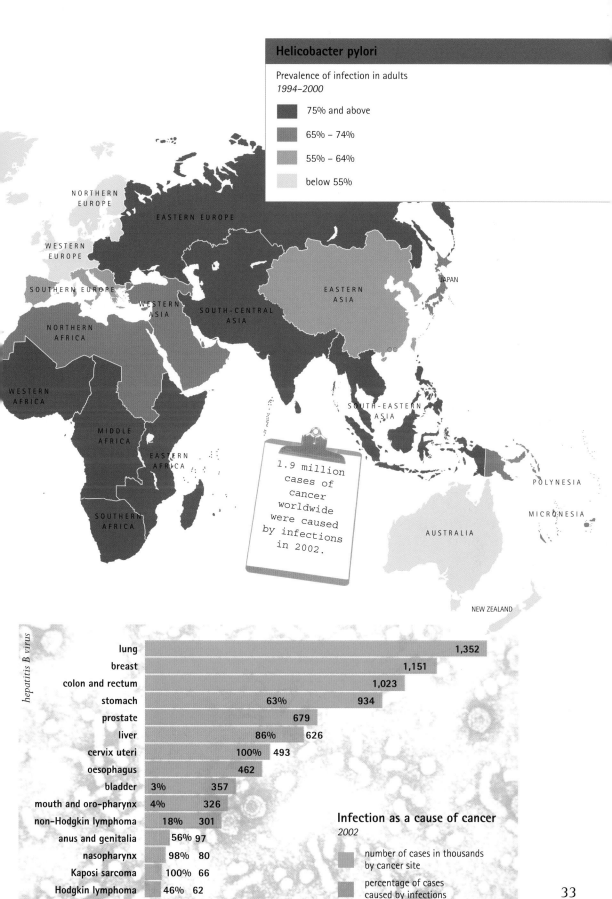

Helicobacter pylori

Prevalence of infection in adults
1994–2000

- 75% and above
- 65% – 74%
- 55% – 64%
- below 55%

NORTHERN
EUROPE

EASTERN EUROPE

WESTERN
EUROPE

SOUTHERN EUROPE

WESTERN
ASIA

SOUTH-CENTRAL
ASIA

EASTERN
ASIA

JAPAN

NORTHERN
AFRICA

WESTERN
AFRICA

MIDDLE
AFRICA

EASTERN
AFRICA

SOUTH-EASTERN
ASIA

SOUTHERN
AFRICA

POLYNESIA

MICRONESIA

AUSTRALIA

NEW ZEALAND

1.9 million
cases of
cancer
worldwide
were caused
by infections
in 2002.

hepatitis B virus

Cancer site	percentage	number of cases (thousands)
lung		1,352
breast		1,151
colon and rectum		1,023
stomach	63%	934
prostate		679
liver	86%	626
cervix uteri	100%	493
oesophagus		462
bladder	3%	357
mouth and oro-pharynx	4%	326
non-Hodgkin lymphoma	18%	301
anus and genitalia	56%	97
nasopharynx	98%	80
Kaposi sarcoma	100%	66
Hodgkin lymphoma	46%	62

Infection as a cause of cancer
2002

- number of cases in thousands
  by cancer site
- percentage of cases
  caused by infections

"He that takes medicine and neglects diet, wastes the skill of the physician."
Chinese proverb

Nutrition, alcohol and physical activity are important influences on cancer risk. Dietary factors account for around 30 percent of cancers in industrialized countries, and 20 percent in developing countries. They may therefore be the most important modifiable cause of cancer. Excess body weight and physical inactivity are estimated to account for between 20 and 33 percent of cancers of the breast (postmenopausal), colon, endometrium, kidney and oesophagus. Alcohol increases the risk of cancers of the head and neck, liver and breast.

Industrialization, urbanization and globalization are resulting in the increased consumption of diets high in fat and low in unrefined carbohydrates. This is combined with a decline in energy expenditure, associated with a more sedentary lifestyle. These changes are leading to chronic diseases, including several cancers (notably breast, colon, prostate, oesophagus) becoming increasingly important causes of disability and death in both developing and newly developed countries, and placing additional burdens on already stretched national health budgets.

While personal lifestyle choices can reduce the risk of cancer, governments and NGOs also have a responsibility to develop food policies conducive to health, create environments friendly to physical activity, and develop interventions targeting children and youth.

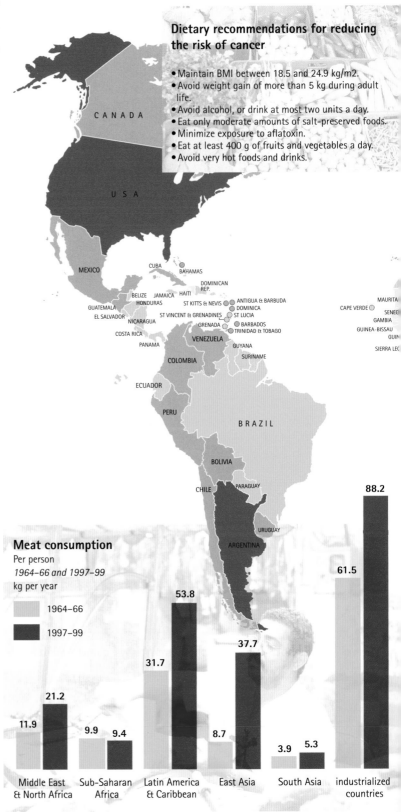

Dietary recommendations for reducing the risk of cancer

- Maintain BMI between 18.5 and 24.9 kg/m2.
- Avoid weight gain of more than 5 kg during adult life.
- Avoid alcohol, or drink at most two units a day.
- Eat only moderate amounts of salt-preserved foods.
- Minimize exposure to aflatoxin.
- Eat at least 400 g of fruits and vegetables a day.
- Avoid very hot foods and drinks.

Meat consumption
Per person
1964–66 and 1997–99
kg per year

- 1964–66
- 1997–99

Region	1964–66	1997–99
Middle East & North Africa	11.9	21.2
Sub-Saharan Africa	9.9	9.4
Latin America & Caribbean	31.7	53.8
East Asia	8.7	37.7
South Asia	3.9	5.3
industrialized countries	61.5	88.2

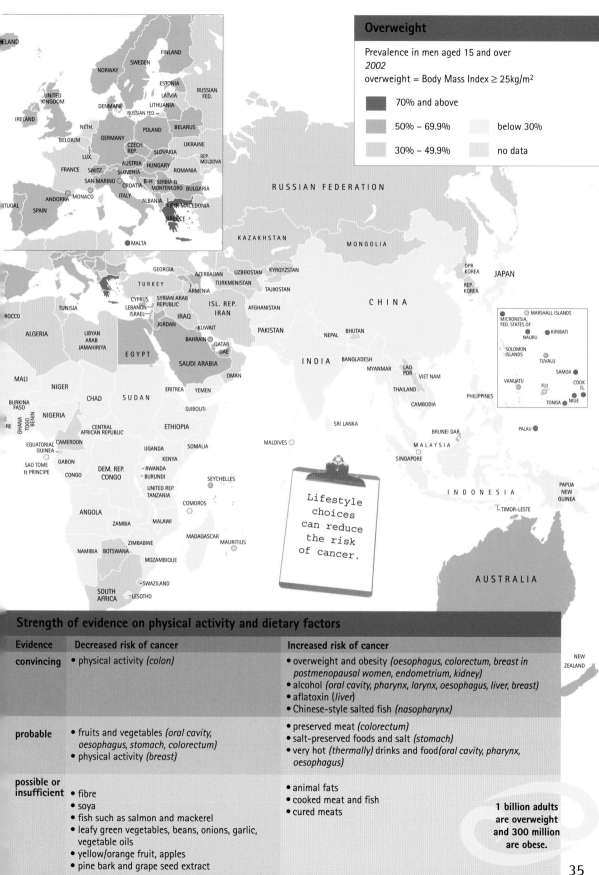

Overweight

Prevalence in men aged 15 and over
2002
overweight = Body Mass Index $\geq$ 25kg/m^2

- 70% and above
- 50% – 69.9%
- 30% – 49.9%
- below 30%
- no data

Lifestyle
choices
can reduce
the risk
of cancer.

1 billion adults
are overweight
and 300 million
are obese.

Strength of evidence on physical activity and dietary factors

Evidence	Decreased risk of cancer	Increased risk of cancer
convincing	• physical activity *(colon)*	• overweight and obesity *(oesophagus, colorectum, breast in postmenopausal women, endometrium, kidney)* • alcohol *(oral cavity, pharynx, larynx, oesophagus, liver, breast)* • aflatoxin *(liver)* • Chinese-style salted fish *(nasopharynx)*
probable	• fruits and vegetables *(oral cavity, oesophagus, stomach, colorectum)* • physical activity *(breast)*	• preserved meat *(colorectum)* • salt-preserved foods and salt *(stomach)* • very hot *(thermally)* drinks and food *(oral cavity, pharynx, oesophagus)*
possible or insufficient	• fibre • soya • fish such as salmon and mackerel • leafy green vegetables, beans, onions, garlic, vegetable oils • yellow/orange fruit, apples • pine bark and grape seed extract	• animal fats • cooked meat and fish • cured meats

The major source of ultraviolet (UV) radiation is the sun. The amount of solar irradiation reaching the Earth's surface depends on latitude, time of day and year, and cloud cover. UV radiation is increasing worldwide with the thinning of the protective ozone layer.

UV radiation causes malignant melanoma of the skin and other skin cancers. The risk depends on skin colour, and type, and is higher if exposure occurs in childhood. The incidence of melanoma is high in countries with pale-skinned populations of European origin and high levels of solar irradiation. The incidence of non-melanoma skin cancers is also very high in these countries, and they are the most frequent type of cancer diagnosed, although very rarely fatal.

Melanoma has shown striking increases in incidence in many white-skinned populations, probably because of increasing recreational exposures to UV. In Europe, the melanoma incidence is highest in the north, not the sunny south, probably because intermittent exposure of pale skin is more important as a cause.

The value of sunscreen in protecting against melanoma is controversial. Sunscreens are only a part of a sun-safe strategy, which includes wearing sunglasses, hats and protective clothing, staying out of the sun at midday, and providing shade structures for outdoor venues.

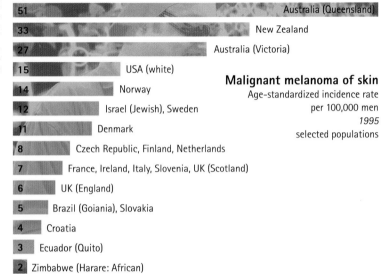

51	Australia (Queensland)
33	New Zealand
27	Australia (Victoria)
15	USA (white)
14	Norway
12	Israel (Jewish), Sweden
11	Denmark
8	Czech Republic, Finland, Netherlands
7	France, Ireland, Italy, Slovenia, UK (Scotland)
6	UK (England)
5	Brazil (Goiania), Slovakia
4	Croatia
3	Ecuador (Quito)
2	Zimbabwe (Harare: African)

Malignant melanoma of skin
Age-standardized incidence rate
per 100,000 men
1995
selected populations

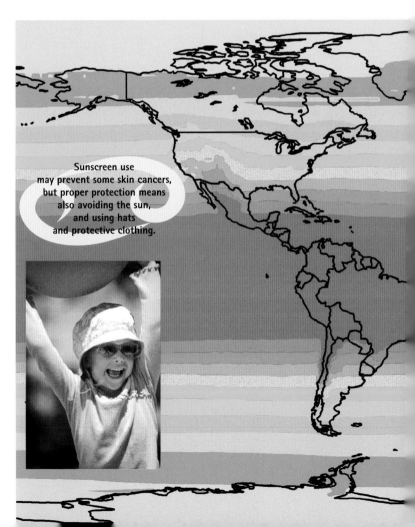

Sunscreen use may prevent some skin cancers, but proper protection means also avoiding the sun, and using hats and protective clothing.

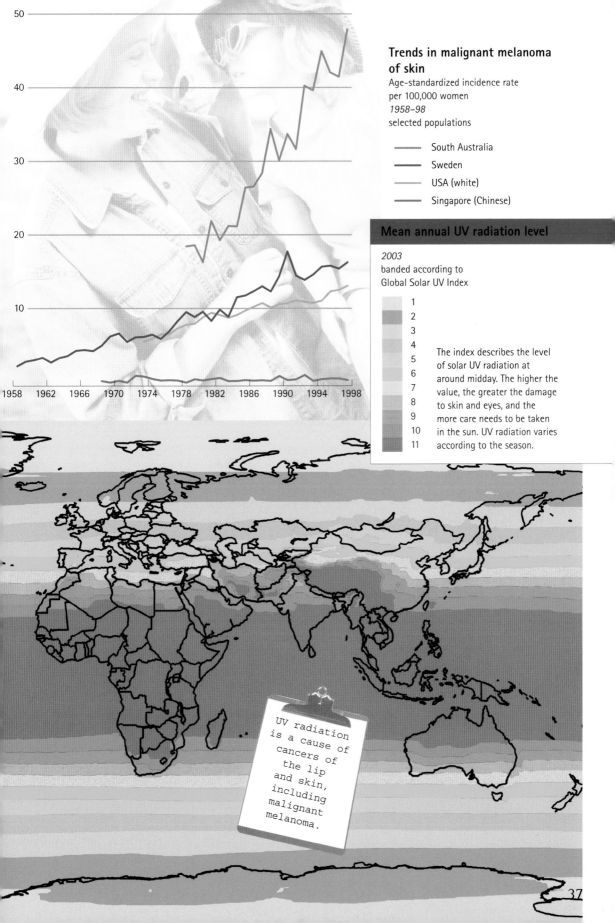

Trends in malignant melanoma of skin
Age-standardized incidence rate
per 100,000 women
1958–98
selected populations

— South Australia
— Sweden
— USA (white)
— Singapore (Chinese)

Mean annual UV radiation level

2003
banded according to
Global Solar UV Index

1
2
3
4
5
6
7
8
9
10
11

The index describes the level of solar UV radiation at around midday. The higher the value, the greater the damage to skin and eyes, and the more care needs to be taken in the sun. UV radiation varies according to the season.

UV radiation is a cause of cancers of the lip and skin, including malignant melanoma.

9 Reproductive and hormonal factors

Reproductive and hormonal factors influence the risk of several cancers of women. Higher rates of breast cancer in developed countries are partly the consequence of women having their first baby later, having fewer pregnancies overall, starting to menstruate earlier and experiencing the menopause later. These changes in risk are related to hormones (mainly oestrogen).

Exposure to exogenous hormones as oral contraceptives and hormone replacement therapy (HRT), results in a small increase in the risk of breast cancer. There is no risk to past users of HRT, and the effect of oral contraceptive use disappears 10 years after cessation. The absolute risk in users of the pill is very small, and easily outweighed by the benefits of effective family planning.

The use of oral contraceptives also slightly increases the risk of cancer of the cervix, but decreases the risk of endometrial and ovarian cancers. The risks of both endometrial cancer and ovarian cancer are increased in women who have neither used hormonal contraception nor had children, while that of cancer of the cervix is increased by childbearing.

A report in 1926 found that breastfeeding was protective against cancer of the breast, an observation confirmed in more recent studies.

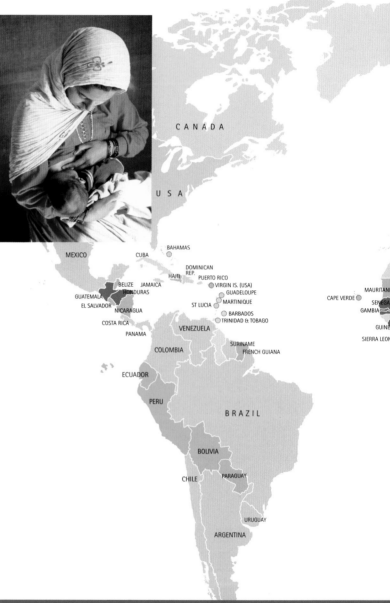

Risk of breast cancer

Increased by:	• oral contraceptives: current users have a risk 24% higher than that of non-users. • hormone replacement therapy: use for 5 years increases risk by 35%.
Decreased by:	• childbearing: risk decreases by 7% for each birth. • breastfeeding: risk declines by 4.3% for each 12 months of breastfeeding.
Not changed by:	• miscarriages. • abortions. • use of HRT or oral contraceptives in the past.

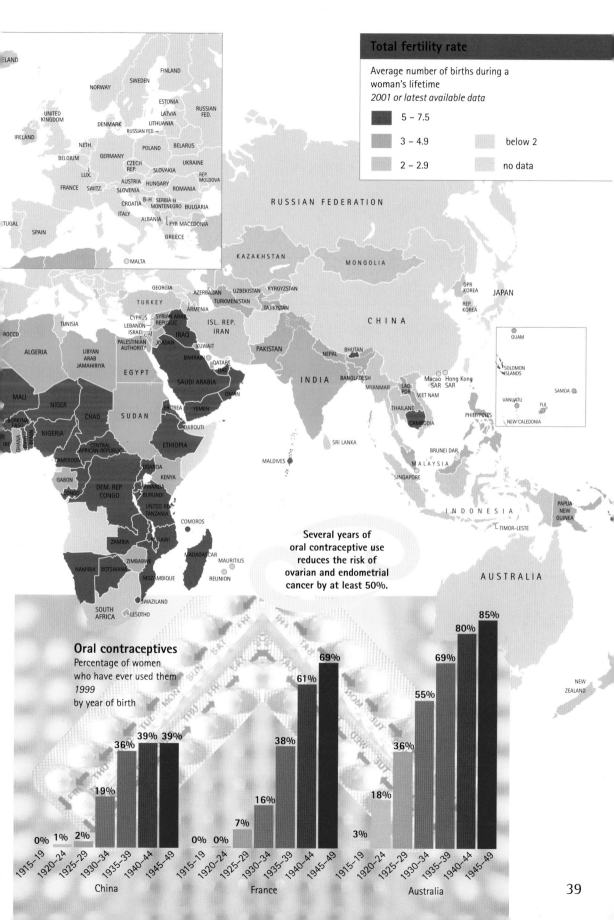

Total fertility rate

Average number of births during a
woman's lifetime
2001 or latest available data

- 5 – 7.5
- 3 – 4.9
- 2 – 2.9
- below 2
- no data

Several years of
oral contraceptive use
reduces the risk of
ovarian and endometrial
cancer by at least 50%.

Oral contraceptives
Percentage of women
who have ever used them
1999
by year of birth

China
- 1915–19: 0%
- 1920–24: 1%
- 1925–29: 2%
- 1930–34: 19%
- 1935–39: 36%
- 1940–44: 39%
- 1945–49: 39%

France
- 1915–19: 0%
- 1920–24: 0%
- 1925–29: 7%
- 1930–34: 16%
- 1935–39: 38%
- 1940–44: 61%
- 1945–49: 69%

Australia
- 1915–19: 3%
- 1920–24: 18%
- 1925–29: 36%
- 1930–34: 55%
- 1935–39: 69%
- 1940–44: 80%
- 1945–49: 85%

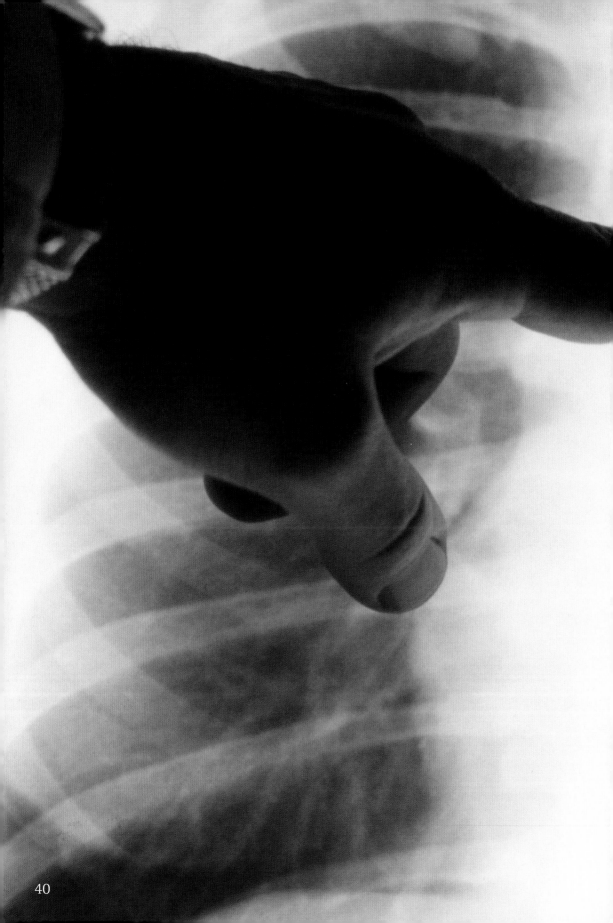

THE BURDEN

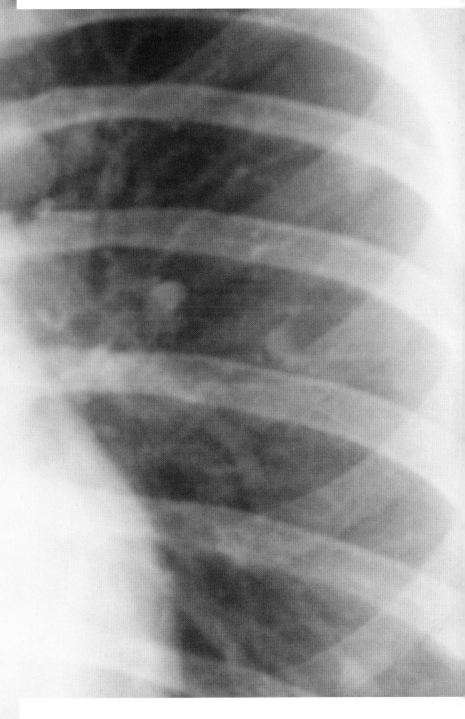

"Before every action ask yourself. Will the result of my action be a blessing or a heavy burden?"

Alfred A Montapert, motivational author, USA

> "One evil in old age is that you think every little illness is the beginning of the end. When a man expects to be arrested, every knock on the door is an alarm."
> Sydney Smith, 1836

The most common cancers involve epithelial tissues (linings of the airways, gastrointestinal and urinary systems), and the risk of these increases rapidly with age, as does the risk of cancer as a whole. Cancer develops when a sequence of mutations occurs in critical genes in one cell of the body, as a result of exposure to carcinogens, such as tobacco, infectious organisms, and chemicals, and internal factors such as inherited mutations, hormones, and immune conditions. Cumulative exposure to such agents increases with time, so that the probability of cancer increases as we age.

In children, certain cancers, such as leukaemias and cancers of connective tissue, are more common than those of epithelial tissues. The risk of cancer is lowest in children aged between 10 and 14 years. Most types of cancer occur more often in men than in women, partly because of greater exposure to carcinogens.

The populations of developing countries are younger than those of the developed regions of the world, and for this reason cancer is less frequent, and the average age at diagnosis is younger than in developed countries. However, the chance of a person developing a cancer during their lifespan does not vary greatly around the world, ranging from about 15 percent by age 65 and 27 percent by age 75 in the USA, compared with 6 percent and 10 percent in Oman.

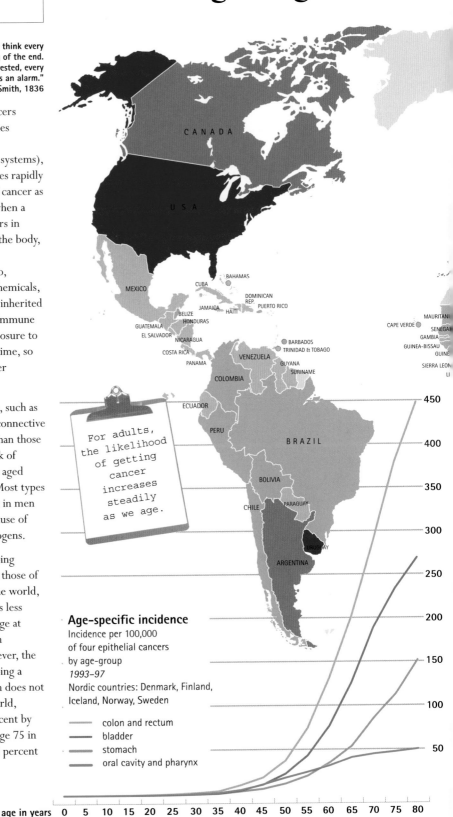

For adults, the likelihood of getting cancer increases steadily as we age.

Age-specific incidence

Incidence per 100,000 of four epithelial cancers by age-group
1993–97
Nordic countries: Denmark, Finland, Iceland, Norway, Sweden

- colon and rectum
- bladder
- stomach
- oral cavity and pharynx

age in years   0   5   10   15   20   25   30   35   40   45   50   55   60   65   70   75   80

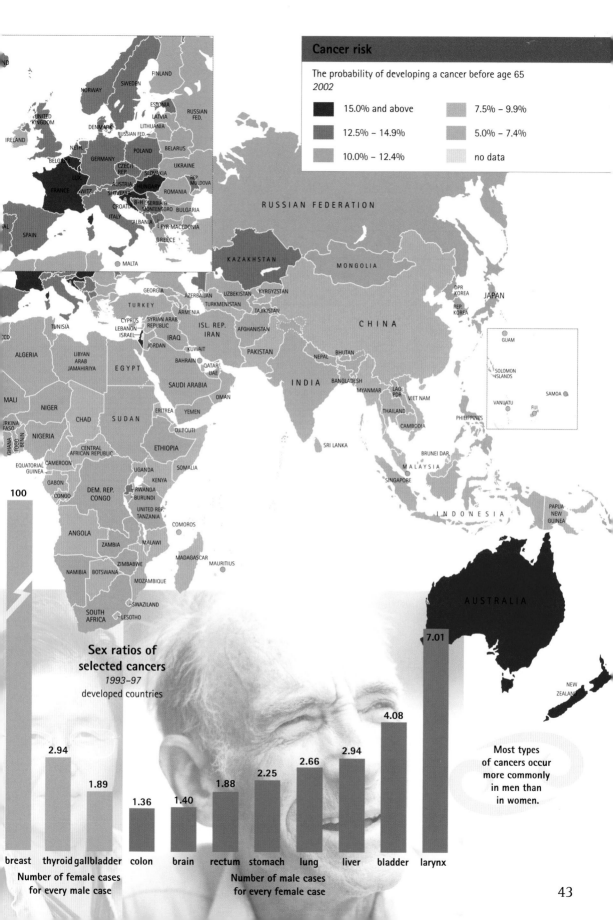

Cancer risk

The probability of developing a cancer before age 65
2002

15.0% and above	7.5% – 9.9%
12.5% – 14.9%	5.0% – 7.4%
10.0% – 12.4%	no data

Sex ratios of selected cancers
1993–97
developed countries

100

2.94

1.89

1.36

1.40

1.88

2.25

2.66

2.94

4.08

7.01

breast   thyroid   gallbladder   colon   brain   rectum   stomach   lung   liver   bladder   larynx

Number of female cases for every male case

Number of male cases for every female case

Most types of cancers occur more commonly in men than in women.

43

In 2002, there were 10.9 million new cancer cases in the world, and 6.7 million deaths. The most common cancers worldwide are lung, breast, large intestine (colon and rectum), stomach and prostate. Liver cancer is the most common cancer for men in several African countries, although Kaposi sarcoma has become the most common in 13 of these countries that are severely affected by the AIDS epidemic. Either breast or cervix cancer is the most common tumour of women in almost all countries (except for some in East Asia, where stomach cancer is more frequent). The cancer that causes the most deaths is lung cancer, followed by stomach and liver cancer, although the pattern is quite different in males and females.

The cancers that are common in developing countries are those that have a poor prognosis (lung, stomach, liver, oesophagus).

Overall, the probability for an individual of dying from cancer during their lifetime is not very different in the developed and developing world.

The risk of getting cancer is higher in the developed world, but cancers in the developing world are more fatal.

Only 19% of the world population live in the developed countries, but 46% of new cancer cases occur there.

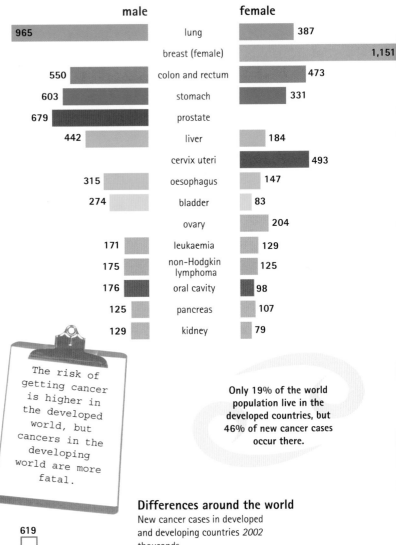

Sex differences
New cancer cases by sex
2002
thousands

male		female
965	lung	387
	breast (female)	1,151
550	colon and rectum	473
603	stomach	331
679	prostate	
442	liver	184
	cervix uteri	493
315	oesophagus	147
274	bladder	83
	ovary	204
171	leukaemia	129
175	non-Hodgkin lymphoma	125
176	oral cavity	98
125	pancreas	107
129	kidney	79

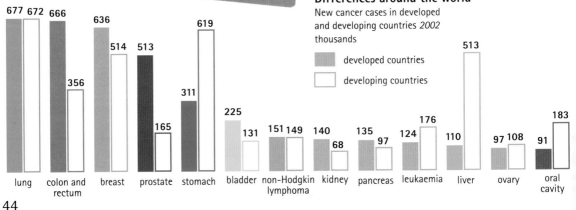

Differences around the world
New cancer cases in developed and developing countries *2002*
thousands

- developed countries
- developing countries

	developed	developing
lung	677	672
colon and rectum	666	356
breast	636	514
prostate	513	165
stomach	311	619
bladder	225	131
non-Hodgkin lymphoma	151	149
kidney	140	68
pancreas	135	97
leukaemia	124	176
liver	110	513
ovary	97	108
oral cavity	91	183

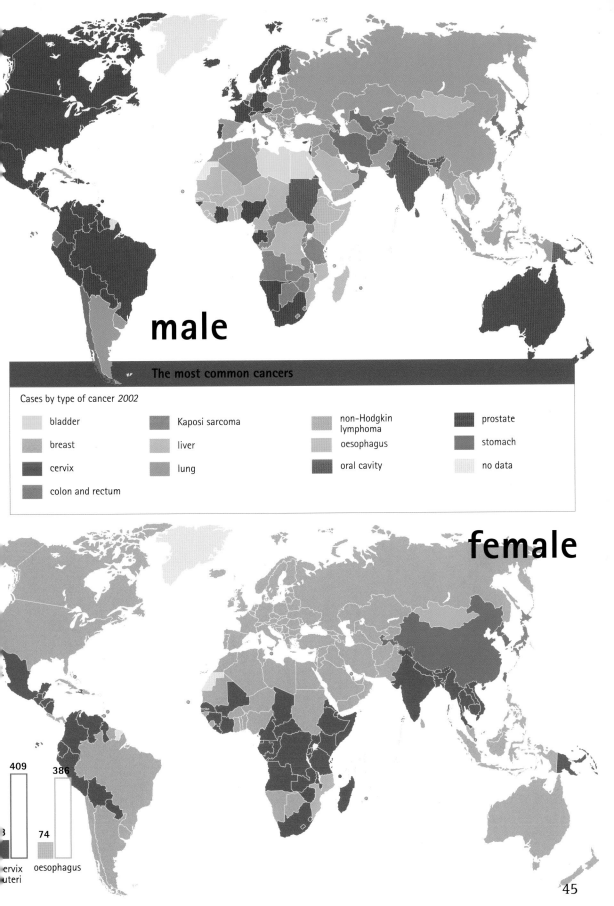

male

The most common cancers

Cases by type of cancer *2002*

- bladder
- breast
- cervix
- colon and rectum
- Kaposi sarcoma
- liver
- lung
- non-Hodgkin lymphoma
- oesophagus
- oral cavity
- prostate
- stomach
- no data

female

409

386

3

74

ervix
uteri

oesophagus

45

Geographical diversity

"You will find, as a general rule, that the constitutions and the habits of a people follow the nature of the land where they live."
Hippocrates (460–370 BCE)

There is a tremendous geographical diversity in the risk of different cancers. Evidence from studies of cancer in migrants, who move from one place of residence to another, confirms that these differences are largely environmental in origin – not due to ethnic or genetic differences – and, especially, a product of different lifestyles.

The pattern of liver cancer reflects the prevalence of infection by hepatitis viruses, especially HBV. One of the main causes of stomach cancer is the bacterium *Helicobacter pylori*. Breast cancer is a disease of affluent countries, but it is not rare anywhere, whereas cervix cancer is largely a disease of the poor south. There are high rates of cancer of the oesophagus in East Africa and Asia, including China and Central Asia, but testis cancer is rare in African and Asian men.

This sort of information shows the priority areas for research, and indicates where implementation of current technology would be most fruitful. The global disparities in incidence of certain preventable cancers (for example, liver and cervix) as well as in survival from several that are treatable (for example, lymphoma, leukaemia and testis) demonstrate a global lack of equity in healthcare. This is apparently determined largely by where one lives.

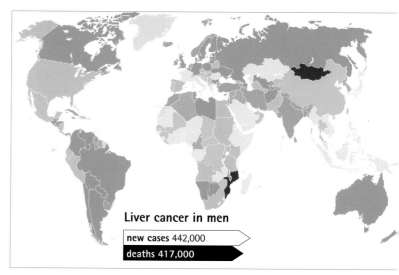

Liver cancer in men

new cases 442,000

deaths 417,000

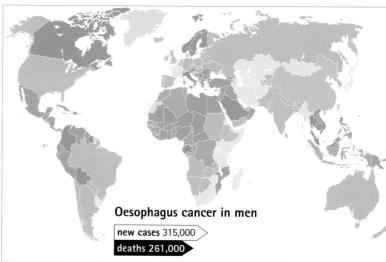

Oesophagus cancer in men

new cases 315,000

deaths 261,000

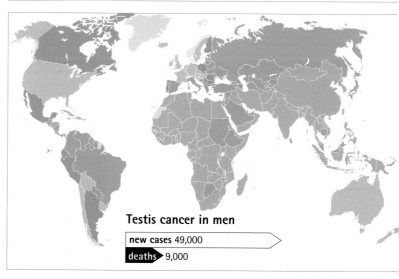

Testis cancer in men

new cases 49,000

deaths 9,000

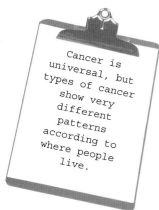

Cancer is universal, but types of cancer show very different patterns according to where people live.

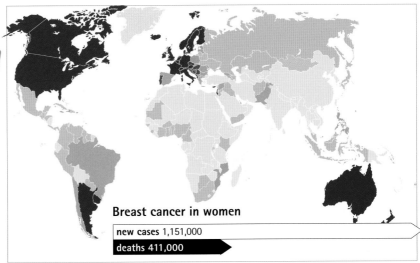

Breast cancer in women

new cases 1,151,000
deaths 411,000

Incidence of cancer

Number of people diagnosed with selected types of cancer
2002
Age-standardized rate per 100,000 people

- 70 and above
- 55 – 69.9
- 40 – 54.9
- 25 – 39.9
- 10 – 24.9
- 5 – 9.9
- 3 – 4.9
- 1 – 2.9
- less than 1
- no data
- new cases *2002*
- deaths *2002*

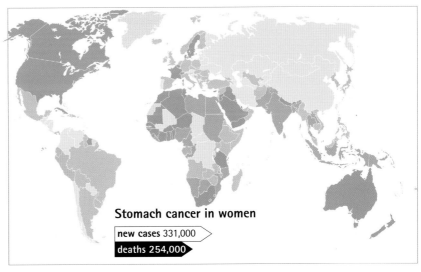

Stomach cancer in women

new cases 331,000
deaths 254,000

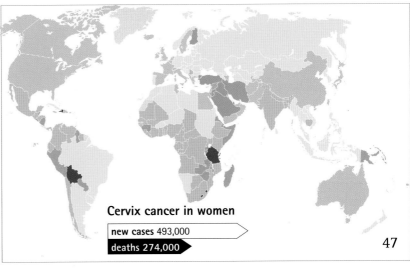

Cervix cancer in women

new cases 493,000
deaths 274,000

47

13 | Lung cancer

Lung cancer is the most common cancer, both in terms of new cases (1.4 million in 2002) and of deaths (1.2 million). Worldwide, about 80 percent of lung cancer cases in men and 50 percent in women are caused by tobacco smoking. Other risk factors include second-hand smoke and exposure to asbestos, radon, arsenic, and air pollution. The younger a person starts smoking, the longer a person smokes, and the more cigarettes a person smokes each day, the greater is the risk of developing lung cancer. All current smokers, regardless of the tar level in their cigarettes, have a substantially greater risk of developing lung cancer than do people who have never smoked or who have quit smoking.

Trends in lung cancer death rates vary widely between countries, according to the stage of the tobacco epidemic. In countries where smoking was first established, the habit has become less common in recent decades, first in men, and later in women, and lung cancer death rates have followed this trend. However, in Eastern and Southern Europe, where tobacco use is still increasing, death rates have climbed in men, and are now rising in women.

Because lung cancer has usually spread by the time of diagnosis, treatment is usually unsuccessful and survival rates are low, with little improvement over time. The key to reducing lung cancer lies in preventing young people from starting to smoke, and encouraging smokers to quit.

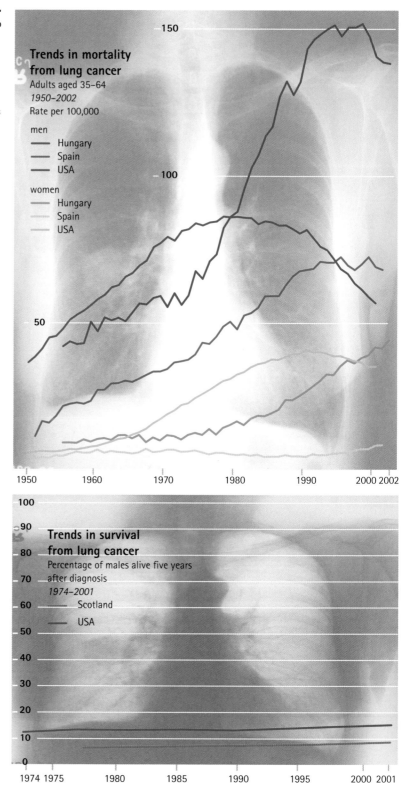

Trends in mortality from lung cancer
Adults aged 35–64
1950–2002
Rate per 100,000

men
— Hungary
— Spain
— USA

women
— Hungary
— Spain
— USA

Trends in survival from lung cancer
Percentage of males alive five years after diagnosis
1974–2001
— Scotland
— USA

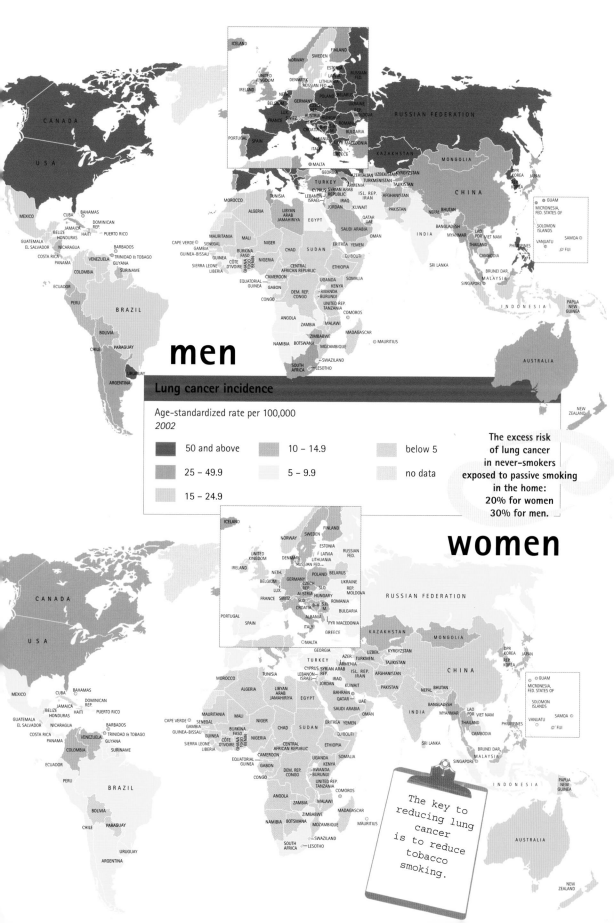

men

Lung cancer incidence

Age-standardized rate per 100,000
2002

- 50 and above
- 25 – 49.9
- 15 – 24.9
- 10 – 14.9
- 5 – 9.9
- below 5
- no data

The excess risk
of lung cancer
in never-smokers
exposed to passive smoking
in the home:
20% for women
30% for men.

women

The key to
reducing lung
cancer
is to reduce
tobacco
smoking.

14 Cancer in children

Cancer is rare in childhood (an estimated 9,510 cases occur in the USA each year), but it is still a leading cause of death in this age group in developed countries.

Acute leukaemia is the most common form of cancer for children in most countries, especially in early childhood. In tropical Africa, lymphomas are more common. Brain tumours generally account for one-fifth to one-quarter of childhood cancers. Carcinomas, the common epithelial cancers of adults, are rare

in children. Sarcomas of bones and soft tissue are much more common, accounting for over 10 percent of cancers, compared with less than 2 percent in adults.

Hereditary cancer syndromes account for the occurrence of several types of childhood cancer (especially retinoblastoma and Wilms tumour). A few environmental exposures have been identified as risk factors, mostly related to infectious agents. These are responsible for the frequency of

Kaposi sarcoma and Burkitt lymphoma in Africa, for example.

There has been an increase in the incidence of childhood cancer in the USA and in Europe since the 1970s, although this may have ceased since the 1990s. However, this has been accompanied by great improvements in the treatment of childhood cancers, with resultant benefits in terms of survival. Mortality from cancer in childhood is therefore falling in the developed world.

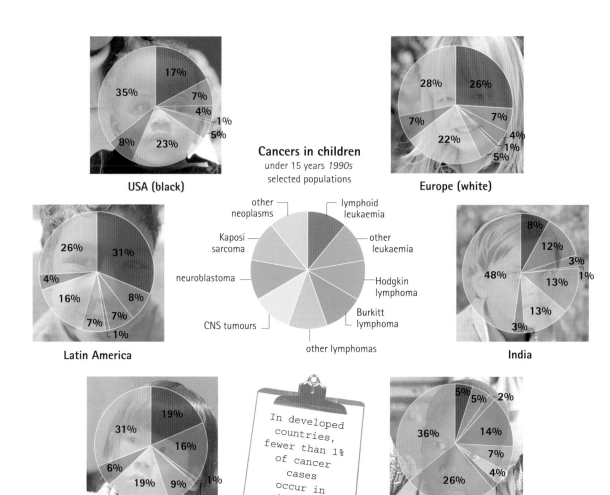

USA (black): 17%, 7%, 4%, 1%, 5%, 23%, 8%, 35%

Europe (white): 28%, 26%, 7%, 7%, 4%, 1%, 5%, 22%

Latin America: 26%, 31%, 4%, 16%, 8%, 7%, 7%, 1%

India: 8%, 12%, 3%, 1%, 13%, 13%, 3%, 48%

East Asia: 19%, 31%, 16%, 6%, 19%, 9%, 1%, <1%

Africa: 5%, 5%, 2%, 36%, 14%, 7%, 4%, 2%, 26%

Cancers in children
under 15 years *1990s*
selected populations

other neoplasms — lymphoid leukaemia
Kaposi sarcoma — other leukaemia
neuroblastoma — Hodgkin lymphoma
CNS tumours — Burkitt lymphoma
other lymphomas

In developed countries, fewer than 1% of cancer cases occur in children.

50   East Asia   Africa

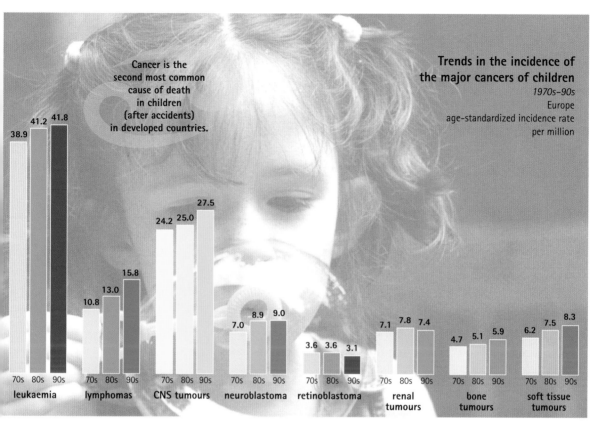

Cancer is the second most common cause of death in children (after accidents) in developed countries.

Trends in the incidence of the major cancers of children
1970s–90s
Europe
age-standardized incidence rate
per million

	70s	80s	90s
leukaemia	38.9	41.2	41.8
lymphomas	10.8	13.0	15.8
CNS tumours	24.2	25.0	27.5
neuroblastoma	7.0	8.9	9.0
retinoblastoma	3.6	3.6	3.1
renal tumours	7.1	7.8	7.4
bone tumours	4.7	5.1	5.9
soft tissue tumours	6.2	7.5	8.3

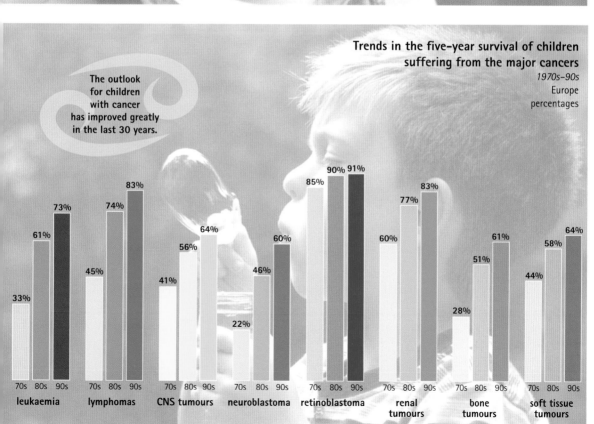

Trends in the five-year survival of children suffering from the major cancers
1970s–90s
Europe
percentages

The outlook for children with cancer has improved greatly in the last 30 years.

	70s	80s	90s
leukaemia	33%	61%	73%
lymphomas	45%	74%	83%
CNS tumours	41%	56%	64%
neuroblastoma	22%	46%	60%
retinoblastoma	85%	90%	91%
renal tumours	60%	77%	83%
bone tumours	28%	51%	61%
soft tissue tumours	44%	58%	64%

51

Cancer survivors

"I don't have any more bad days. I have good days and I have great days. Cancer no longer consumes my life, my thoughts, or my behaviour."
Lance Armstrong,
cancer survivor and champion cyclist

Cancer survivors are people who have been diagnosed with cancer at some point in their lives. Family and friends are also affected by a diagnosis of cancer, and thus are, in a way, survivors too.

Worldwide, in 2002, there were approximately 24.6 million cancer survivors who had been diagnosed within the previous 5 years. That number will increase steadily during the coming years, as the average age of the world's population increases.

Variations in the proportion of cancer survivors in a population are related to a number of factors: the age distribution of the population; the types of cancer occurring; the incidence rates of each; the amount of cancer screening and early detection; the proportion of patients who receive effective cancer treatment; and rates of death from other causes.

Survivors may face numerous physical, psychological and financial challenges throughout the remainder of their lives. Effective treatment is the most important strategy to ensure optimal life following a cancer diagnosis. However, there are many other interventions that can improve a survivor's life. Unfortunately, access to these interventions is not available equally around the world. Efforts such as Relay For Life help to raise funds and awareness in support of survivors. Additional resources are needed to help the millions of cancer survivors worldwide.

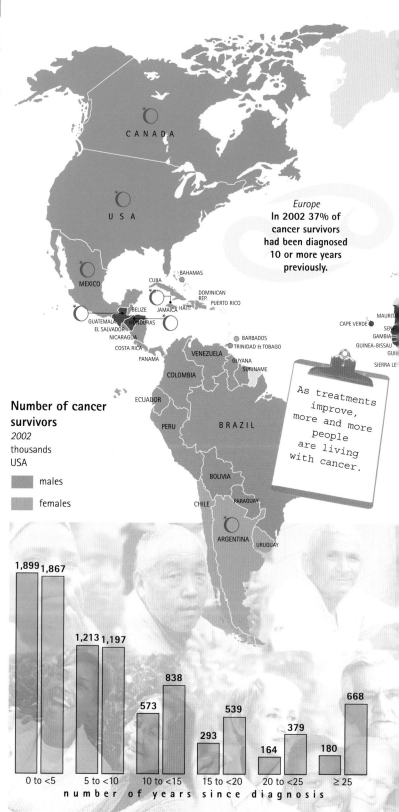

Europe
In 2002 37% of cancer survivors had been diagnosed 10 or more years previously.

As treatments improve, more and more people are living with cancer.

Number of cancer survivors
2002
thousands
USA

- males
- females

number of years since diagnosis	males	females
0 to <5	1,899	1,867
5 to <10	1,213	1,197
10 to <15	573	838
15 to <20	293	539
20 to <25	164	379
≥ 25	180	668

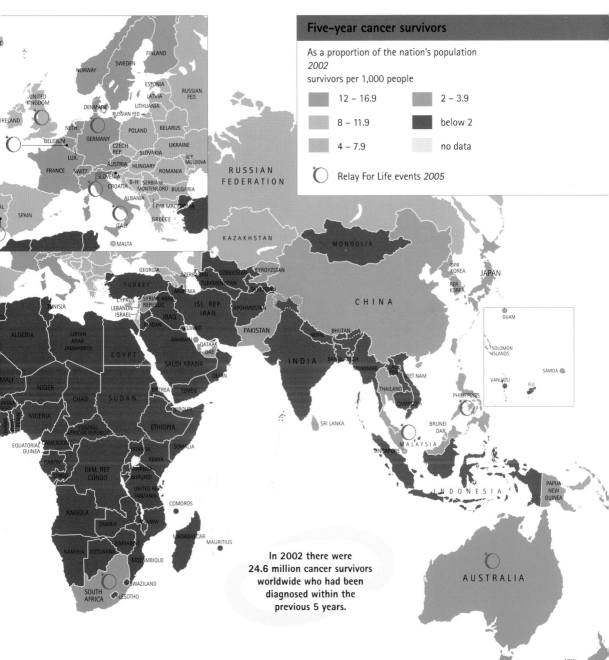

Five-year cancer survivors

As a proportion of the nation's population
2002
survivors per 1,000 people

12 – 16.9	2 – 3.9
8 – 11.9	below 2
4 – 7.9	no data

◯ Relay For Life events *2005*

RUSSIAN
FEDERATION

In 2002 there were
24.6 million cancer survivors
worldwide who had been
diagnosed within the
previous 5 years.

Relay For Life

Relay For Life are community events around the world that bring together people who share the common goals of eliminating cancer and celebrating surviving cancer. Volunteers form teams that make a commitment to raise money through individual and team events. At an event, relay teams take turns walking or running around a track or path. Each team keeps at least one representative on the track at all times, during a relay that lasts up to 24 hours. During the event, local entertainers perform, and families enjoy fun activities.

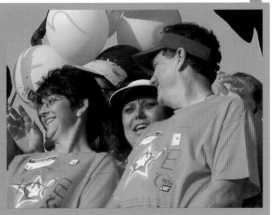

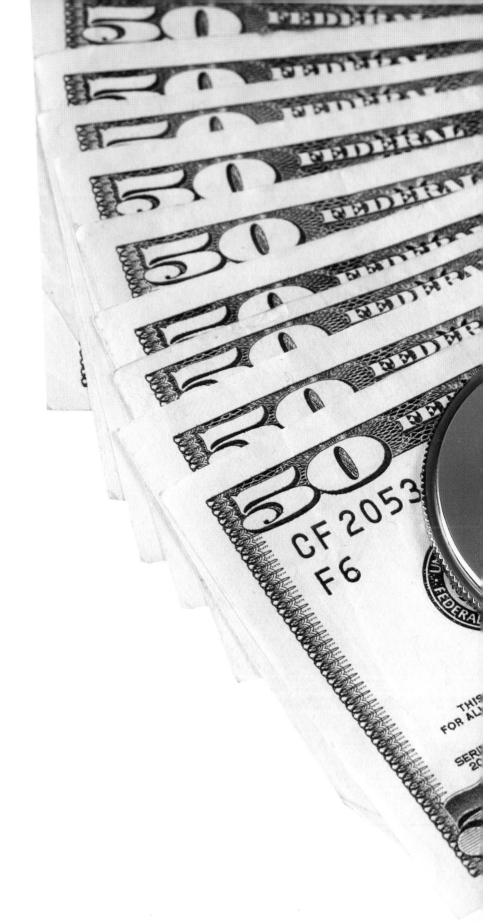

PART FOUR

ECONOMICS

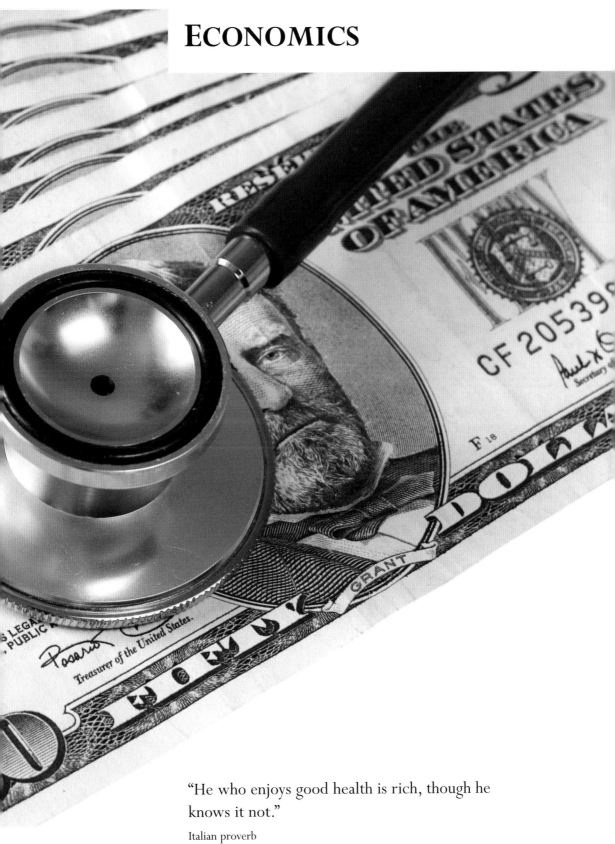

"He who enjoys good health is rich, though he knows it not."

Italian proverb

"Economics is first and foremost about the thoughts leading up to choice."
Gerald P O'Driscoll, Former Director, Center for International Trade and Economics, Heritage Foundation

The costs of cancer are quite diverse. First, the direct costs include payments and resources used for treatment, care and rehabilitation directly related to the illness. Indirect costs include the loss of economic output due to days off work (morbidity costs) and premature death (mortality costs). There are also the hidden costs of cancer, such as health insurance premiums and non-medical expenses (for example, transportation, child or elder care, housekeeping assistance, wigs, ostomy supplies, prostheses). Cancer prevention may be the best way to save money for many countries as these costs continue to rise.

Data limitations do not allow for a worldwide comparison of the economic costs of cancer; these data only represent selected countries.

USA and Canada

The total cost of cancer in the USA in 2005 was US$209.9 billion. US spending on cancer care has dramatically increased yet its proportion of health expenditures has remained virtually constant.

Use of the new drugs Avastin and Eloxatin has doubled survival rates for metastatic colorectal cancer, while increasing treatment costs by 500-fold.

In 1998, the cost of treating cancer in Canada was US$14.2 billion (9% of all disease costs, ranking third).

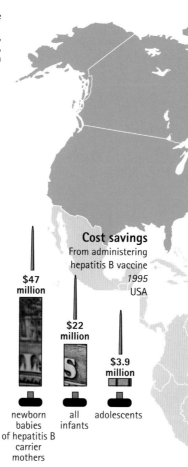

Cost savings
From administering hepatitis B vaccine
1995
USA

$47 million — newborn babies of hepatitis B carrier mothers

$22 million — all infants

$3.9 million — adolescents

The cost of treating obesity
As a percentage of all adult health expenditure
2003
USA

6% (US$75 billion)

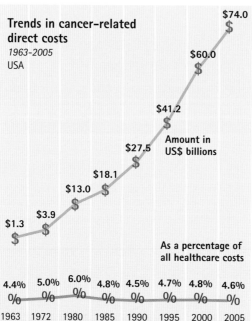

Trends in cancer-related direct costs
1963-2005
USA

Amount in US$ billions

$1.3
$3.9
$13.0
$18.1
$27.5
$41.2
$60.0
$74.0

Chile

Treatment for tobacco-related lung cancer accounted for 6% of total healthcare costs in 2004.

As a percentage of all healthcare costs

1963	1972	1980	1985	1990	1995	2000	2005
4.4%	5.0%	6.0%	4.8%	4.5%	4.7%	4.8%	4.6%

The cost of breast cancer treatment

Cost per patient of first 6 months of treatment
expressed as percentage of GDP per capita
published 2003 or latest available data
selected countries

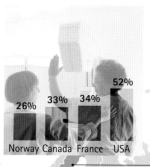

26% Norway
33% Canada
34% France
52% USA

Sweden

Total cancer drug sales rose from
US$37.3 million in 2000 to
US$118.7 million in 2004.

UK

Expenditure on cancer
treatment by the National
Health Service in 2000-01
was US$3.2 billion (10.6% of
all disease costs).

The Netherlands

In 1999, the cost of cancer care
was US$1.2 billion. The cost of
smoking-related healthcare for
those aged 20 years and older
was US$514 million.

**Smoking
accounts for 6%-15% of
annual healthcare costs
in high-income
countries.**

France

Cancer hospitalizations
within the public health
system cost US$6.2
billion in 1999 (23% for
chemotherapy).

Estimated total cancer
drug sales in 2002 were
US$1.3-1.6 billion.

Switzerland

The Benefit-Cost Ratio for
hepatitis B vaccinations in 1998
was 2.4 for vaccinating all
infants, 1.2 for vaccinating
newborns of hepatitis B carrier
mothers, and 2.9 for
vaccinating all adolescents.
(*Values greater than 1.0 indicate
net savings.*)

China

The Benefit-Cost Ratio for hepatitis
B vaccinations in 1995 was 42.4 –
48.0 for vaccinating all infants.
(*Values greater than 1.0 indicate net
savings.*)

**Cigarettes
are most affordable in
high-income countries,
even when prices increase
with tobacco taxes.**

**The costs of
cancer pose an
economic
burden on both
the individual
and society.**

The price of 100 packs of cigarettes

As a percentage of GDP per capita
1999-2001
selected countries

Country	%
Luxembourg	0.4%
Japan	0.6%
France	1.1%
Bahrain	1.2%
Canada	1.3%
Hungary	1.7%
Brazil	2.4%
Russian Federation	3.2%
Turkey	3.7%
South Africa	4.5%
Morocco	11.3%
China	19.2%
India	21.4%
Bangladesh	23.2%
Nigeria	29.8%

17 | Commercial interests

Industries make a vital contribution to relieving the cancer burden. Their role is not just research and development; probably more important is their role in manufacture, marketing, and distribution of existing and new pharmaceuticals and technology products. There are few instances where governments or non-profit organisations take on these latter functions.

Businesses also provide benefits to employees and their families related to cancer control, such as underwriting health insurance and instituting workplace prevention programmes (smoking cessation, fitness centres, healthy food choices). Private businesses provide financial support to the prevention and treatment of cancer, as part of their social responsibility programmes – these include examples that range from the cosmetic industry to restaurant chains.

Yet, commercial activities sometimes contribute to causing cancer, through the side-effects of their products, or by the creation of unsafe environments in or around the workplace. The best-known example is the tobacco industry, which ranks among the most powerful commercial enterprises, and which also owns other major industries such as food companies. Revelations from internal tobacco industry documents are clear: the tobacco industry has consistently lied or obscured the truth about the harmfulness – including the cancer risk – and addictive nature of tobacco. In addition, carcinogenic substances encountered at work include asbestos, arsenic, benzene, silica and secondhand tobacco smoke.

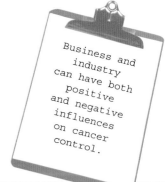

Business and industry can have both positive and negative influences on cancer control.

Some of the industries that contribute to the prevention, diagnosis and treatment of cancer

Industry	Examples of products for cancer control
pharmaceutical	• smoking-cessation gum or patch • vaccines for cancer prevention • drugs to treat cancers
medical supply	• intravenous pumps • central venous ports • radioactive materials • feeding tubes • ostomy bags
rehabilitation	• limb prosthetics • visual aids
equipment	• wheelchairs • breast implants
biotechnology	• artificial bone • tests for cancer genes • DNA probes
medical devices	• radiotherapy • imaging (mammography, ultrasound, CT scans) • colonoscopes

Biomedical research

Funding in USA by source 2003

government: $37.6 billion

industry: $54.1 billion

- medical device firms 10%
- biotechnology firms 19%
- National Institutes of Health 28%
- pharmaceutical firms 29%
- other federal funding 7%
- state and local government 5%
- foundations, charities and other private funds 3% $2.5 billion

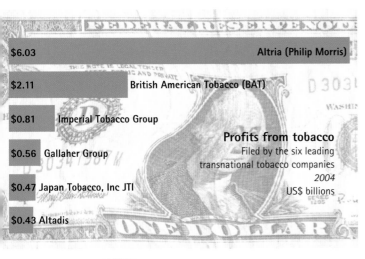

$6.03	Altria (Philip Morris)
$2.11	British American Tobacco (BAT)
$0.81	Imperial Tobacco Group
$0.56	Gallaher Group
$0.47	Japan Tobacco, Inc JTI
$0.43	Altadis

Profits from tobacco
Filed by the six leading
transnational tobacco companies
2004
US$ billions

About 1 in every 5
cancer deaths worldwide
is caused by tobacco.

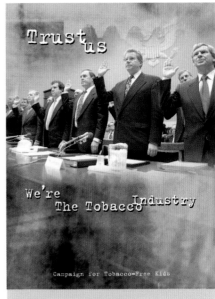

USA
US Congressional Hearing, House of
Representatives, 1994.
Senior tobacco industry executives swear
under oath that nicotine is not addictive.
(Campaign for Tobacco-Free Kids, Ash UK
publication)

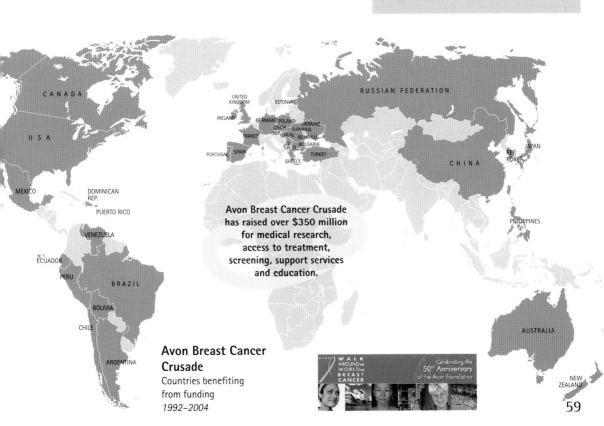

Avon Breast Cancer Crusade
has raised over $350 million
for medical research,
access to treatment,
screening, support services
and education.

**Avon Breast Cancer
Crusade**
Countries benefiting
from funding
1992–2004

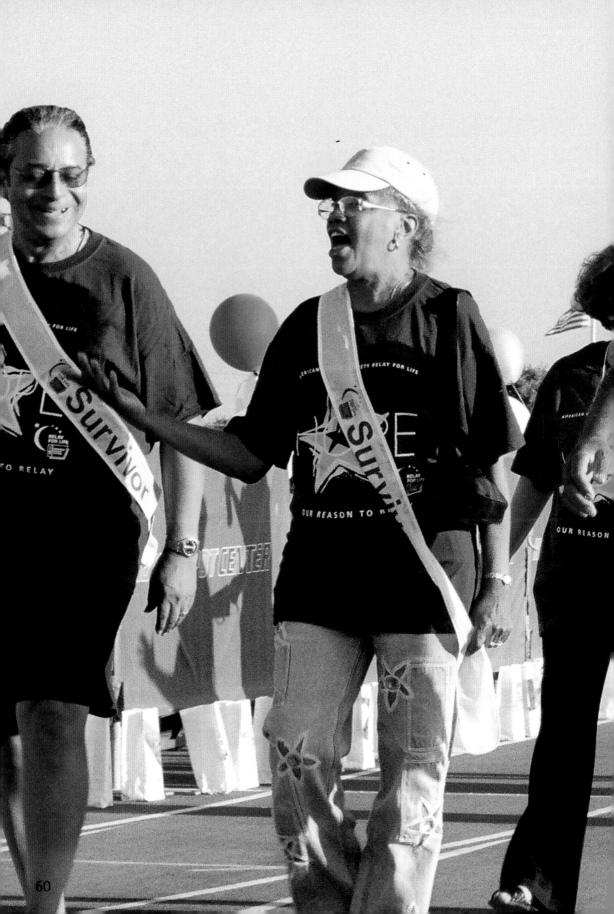

PART FIVE

TAKING ACTION

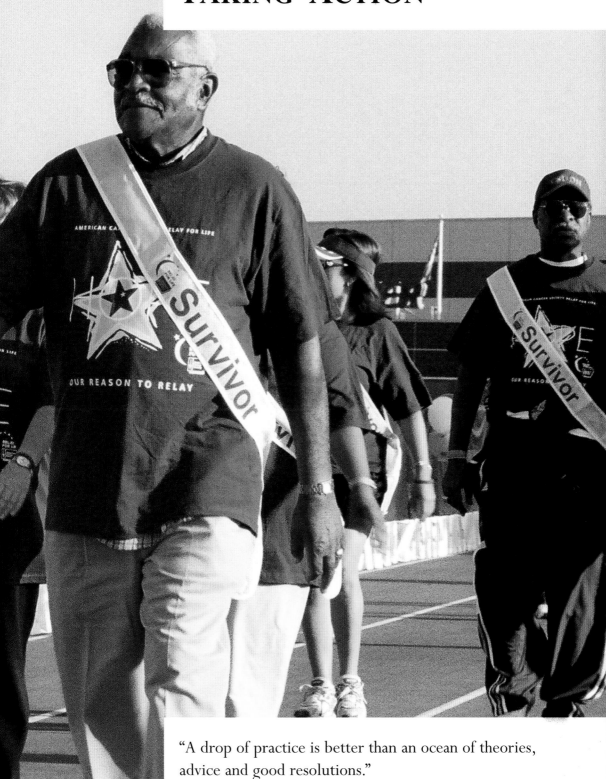

"A drop of practice is better than an ocean of theories, advice and good resolutions."

Sri Aurobindo Society of Hong Kong, 2005

18 | Cancer registries

Cancer registries collect details of new cancer cases, and their follow up, either for a defined population (usually a geographical area) or for a hospital. They provide detailed information about cancer patients, the nature of their tumour (including the precise histological type, and stage of disease), treatment received, and the outcome of the disease.

Population-based cancer registries produce statistics on cancer incidence, mortality and survival, and have public health and research functions. Statistics on cancer risk and outcome in the population, and their changes over time, are essential in planning and evaluating cancer control programmes. Cancer registries are also widely used in cancer research studies for tracing cancer cases and following them up.

The first such registries (Hamburg in Germany, Connecticut in the USA, and in Denmark) were established more than 60 years ago. Cancer registries may cover entire national populations, or, for larger countries, more usually the component regions, states or provinces. Several regional associations exist for sharing experience and methodology. The International Association of Cancer Registries (IACR), founded in 1966, has a global membership, and sponsors a variety of publications, including, every five years, in collaboration with IARC, *Cancer Incidence in Five Continents*, which contains statistical data from all the best-quality registries worldwide.

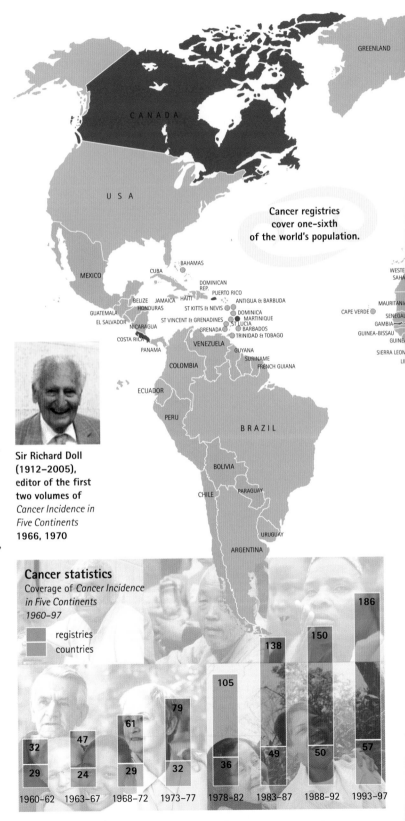

Cancer registries cover one-sixth of the world's population.

Sir Richard Doll (1912–2005), editor of the first two volumes of *Cancer Incidence in Five Continents* **1966, 1970**

Cancer statistics
Coverage of *Cancer Incidence in Five Continents* *1960–97*

- registries
- countries

	1960–62	1963–67	1968–72	1973–77	1978–82	1983–87	1988–92	1993–97
registries	32	47	61	79	105	138	150	186
countries	29	24	29	32	36	49	50	57

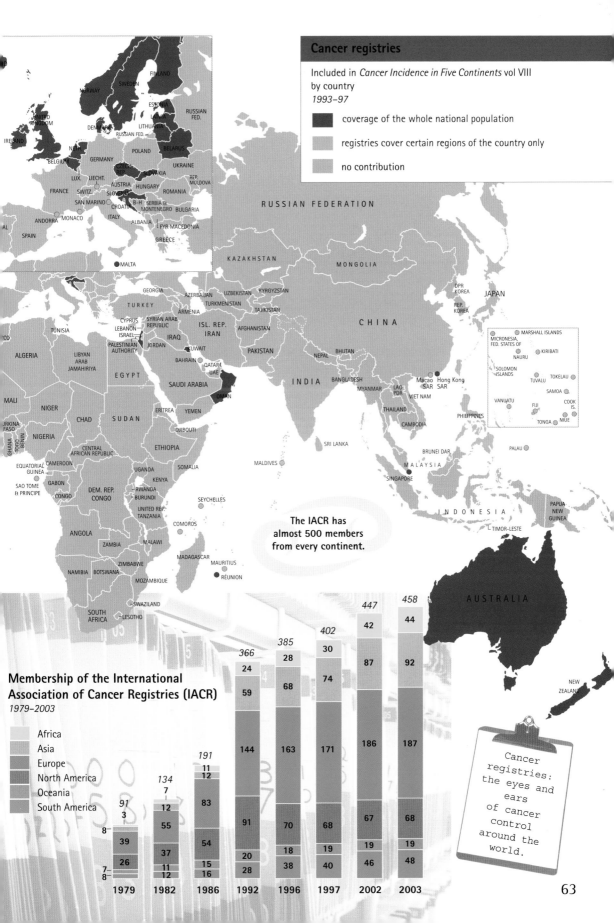

Cancer registries

Included in *Cancer Incidence in Five Continents* vol VIII
by country
1993–97

- coverage of the whole national population
- registries cover certain regions of the country only
- no contribution

The IACR has almost 500 members from every continent.

Cancer registries: the eyes and ears of cancer control around the world.

Membership of the International Association of Cancer Registries (IACR)
1979–2003

- Africa
- Asia
- Europe
- North America
- Oceania
- South America

	1979	1982	1986	1992	1996	1997	2002	2003
Total	91	134	191	366	385	402	447	458
South America	3	7	11	24	28	30	42	44
Oceania	8	12	12	59	68	74	87	92
North America	39	55	83	144	163	171	186	187
Europe	26	37	54	91	70	68	67	68
Asia	7	11	15	20	18	19	19	19
Africa	8	12	16	28	38	40	46	48

63

19 | Research

From the description of how a cancer cell works to the elucidation of the human genome, scientific advances in basic, clinical, and population-based cancer research, and their global impact, have been phenomenal. Recent developments have made available new and improved treatments that have both increased survival and decreased toxicity.

International collaborative efforts for cancer research have substantially increased. This has become the focus of organizations such as the International Network for Cancer Treatment and Research, International Agency for Research on Cancer, US National Cancer Institute, International Cancer Research Portfolio partners, and Bill and Melinda Gates Foundation. A tremendous expansion of the cancer research and development industry has led to a massive increase in spending by for-profit entities such as pharmaceutical companies.

Despite these improvements, several challenges still remain. Developed countries must assure proper translation of cancer research into everyday clinical and public health practice. Developing countries should focus on building the capacity for research through collaborative projects that incorporate localized training and educational programmes. Scientists should focus on increasing the quantity and quality of research that provides knowledge about diverse populations and environments around the world. Additionally, the substantial worldwide disparity in research activities and funding needs to be addressed.

Funding in USA

Grants, contracts and research conducted at the US National Institutes of Health *2004*
US$ millions

$5,547	cancer
$4,911	neurosciences
$3,055	infectious diseases
$2,360	cardiovascular disease
$1,818	mental health
$1,629	biodefense
$996	diabetes
$536	tobacco
$513	infant mortality
$422	obesity
$378	hypertension

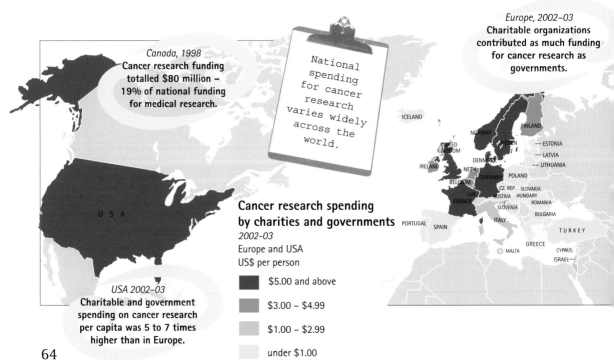

Canada, 1998
Cancer research funding totalled $80 million – 19% of national funding for medical research.

National spending for cancer research varies widely across the world.

USA 2002–03
Charitable and government spending on cancer research per capita was 5 to 7 times higher than in Europe.

Europe, 2002–03
Charitable organizations contributed as much funding for cancer research as governments.

ICELAND, NORWAY, FINLAND, UNITED KINGDOM, SWEDEN, ESTONIA, LATVIA, DENMARK, LITHUANIA, IRELAND, NETH, GERMANY, POLAND, BELGIUM, LUX, CZ. REP., SLOVAKIA, AUSTRIA, HUNGARY, FRANCE, SLOVENIA, ROMANIA, ITALY, BULGARIA, PORTUGAL, SPAIN, TURKEY, GREECE, MALTA, CYPRUS, ISRAEL

Cancer research spending by charities and governments
2002-03
Europe and USA
US$ per person

- $5.00 and above
- $3.00 – $4.99
- $1.00 – $2.99
- under $1.00

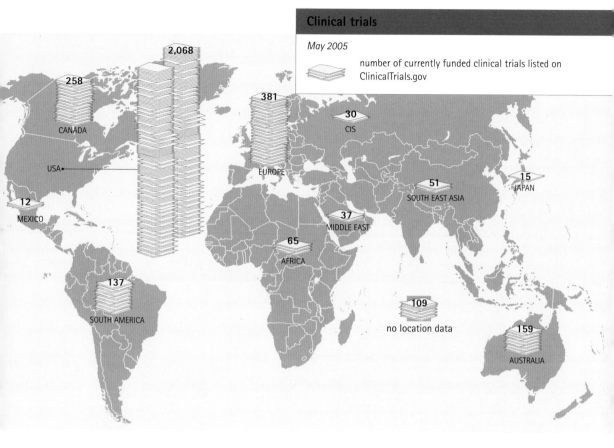

Clinical trials

May 2005

number of currently funded clinical trials listed on ClinicalTrials.gov

258 CANADA

2,068

USA

12 MEXICO

137 SOUTH AMERICA

381 EUROPE

30 CIS

37 MIDDLE EAST

65 AFRICA

51 SOUTH EAST ASIA

15 JAPAN

109 no location data

159 AUSTRALIA

Studies in the International Cancer Research Portfolio database

Number in each research category
2004–05

Total: 21,713 studies

Europe & USA, 2002–03
Less than 10% of cancer research funding was allocated to prevention.

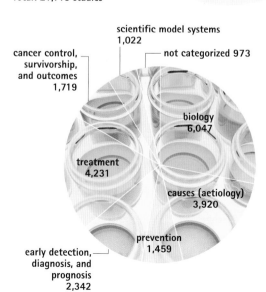

scientific model systems
1,022

not categorized 973

cancer control, survivorship, and outcomes
1,719

biology
6,047

treatment
4,231

causes (aetiology)
3,920

early detection, diagnosis, and prognosis
2,342

prevention
1,459

Study protocols of the European Organization for Research and Treatment of Cancer

Number of protocols by treatment type
July 2005

Total: 752

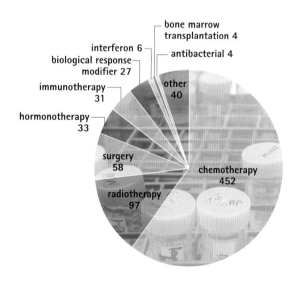

bone marrow transplantation 4

interferon 6

antibacterial 4

biological response modifier 27

immunotherapy
31

other
40

hormonotherapy
33

surgery
58

chemotherapy
452

radiotherapy
97

65

Tobacco use, alcohol consumption, being overweight or obese and physical inactivity play major roles in the development of cancer. These modifiable risk factors contribute to about two-thirds of all cancers in western countries and at least one-third throughout the world.

The worldwide cancer burden is projected to grow as people in developing countries live longer and increasingly adopt western lifestyles, including higher consumption of saturated fat and calorie-dense foods, and reduced physical activity at work and during leisure time.

About 27 percent of cancers in developing countries and 18 percent worldwide are related to infection. Some of these are preventable through immunization; vaccination against hepatitis B (to prevent liver cancer) is well established, while a vaccine against the human papilloma virus (the cause of cancer of the cervix) is being developed. Anti-retroviral treatment can reduce the risk of AIDS-related cancers in HIV-infected subjects.

Pharmacologic agents can also be useful in cancer prevention (tamoxifen and raloxifene for chemoprevention of breast cancer in high-risk women). Primary prevention efforts that promote smoking cessation, reduction of adolescent smoking, healthy eating habits, physical activity, and UV protection should have high priority in cancer control programmes.

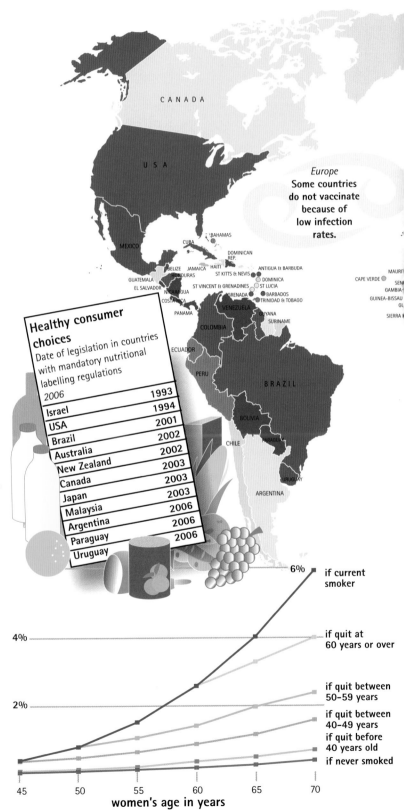

Europe
Some countries do not vaccinate because of low infection rates.

Healthy consumer choices
Date of legislation in countries with mandatory nutritional labelling regulations

2006	1993
Israel	1994
USA	2001
Brazil	2002
Australia	2002
New Zealand	2003
Canada	2003
Japan	2003
Malaysia	2006
Argentina	2006
Paraguay	2006
Uruguay	

6% — if current smoker

4% — if quit at 60 years or over

if quit between 50–59 years

2% — if quit between 40–49 years
if quit before 40 years old
if never smoked

45   50   55   60   65   70
women's age in years

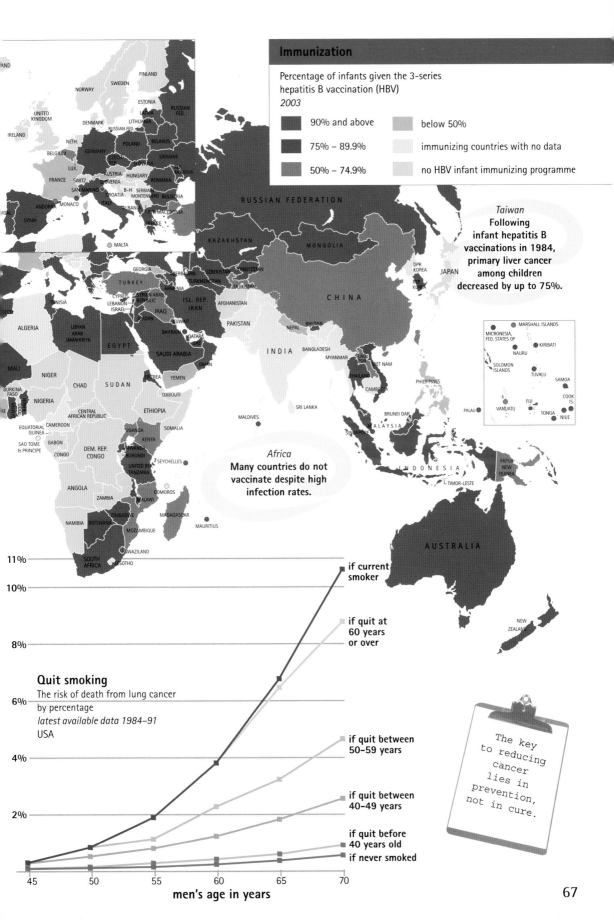

Percentage of infants given the 3-series
hepatitis B vaccination (HBV)
2003

■	90% and above	■ below 50%
■	75% – 89.9%	■ immunizing countries with no data
■	50% – 74.9%	■ no HBV infant immunizing programme

Taiwan
**Following
infant hepatitis B
vaccinations in 1984,
primary liver cancer
among children
decreased by up to 75%.**

Africa
**Many countries do not
vaccinate despite high
infection rates.**

Quit smoking

The risk of death from lung cancer
by percentage
latest available data 1984–91
USA

if current
smoker

if quit at
60 years
or over

if quit between
50–59 years

if quit between
40–49 years

if quit before
40 years old

if never smoked

men's age in years

The key
to reducing
cancer
lies in
prevention,
not in cure.

67

Prevention: population and systems approaches

"The health of the people is really the foundation upon which all their happiness and all their powers as a state depend."
Benjamin Disraeli, Prime Minister (1804–81)

Cancer prevention programmes are being increasingly linked to reductions in incidence and/or mortality. These programmes either simply encourage healthy behaviour changes, or focus on policies that support such changes (for example tobacco taxes, nutritional advice, shade structures, immunization). Childhood hepatocellular carcinoma incidence in Taiwan has substantially decreased since the introduction of a national policy for universal infant hepatitis B vaccination. Anti-smoking campaigns in many industrialized nations have resulted in considerable decreases in smoking-related cancer mortality. Nationwide skin-cancer programmes in Australia (which began in the 1980s and are now recognized as the most comprehensive, well funded, and longest lasting of any others worldwide) have successfully produced changes in sun protection attitudes and behaviours.

The success of national cancer prevention initiatives depends on compliance amongst the target population, but to an even greater extent on a country's health services infrastructure. There is much global variation in the resources necessary for cancer control, including equipment, facilities, funding, and trained medical professionals. To achieve the most impact, national authorities must select activities that make the most efficient use of resources and are acceptable and relevant to society.

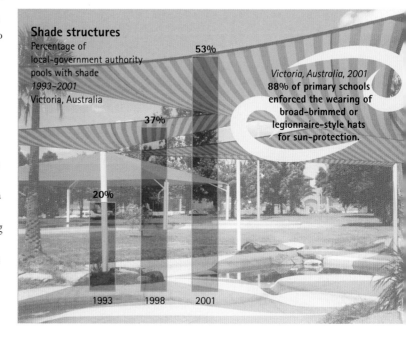

Shade structures
Percentage of local-government authority pools with shade
1993–2001
Victoria, Australia

53%

37%

20%

1993　　1998　　2001

Victoria, Australia, 2001
88% of primary schools enforced the wearing of broad-brimmed or legionnaire-style hats for sun-protection.

Effectiveness of measures to prevent smoking in young people
Decreases in prevalence of youth smoking after anti-tobacco campaigns
1999–2002, 2000–03

prevalence before campaign

prevalence after campaign

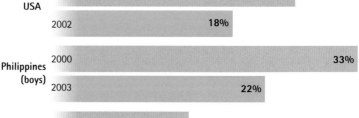

USA	1999	25%
	2002	18%
Philippines (boys)	2000	33%
	2003	22%
Philippines (girls)	2000	13%
	2003	9%

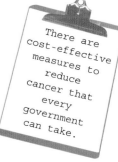

There are cost-effective measures to reduce cancer that every government can take.

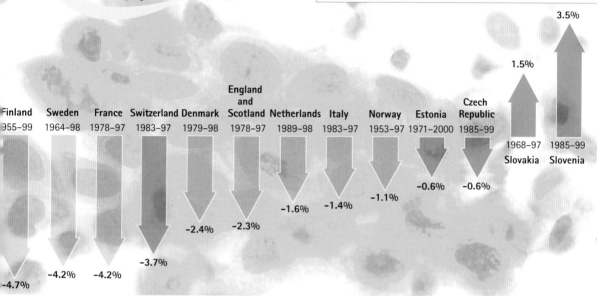

Europe
Marked declines in the incidence of invasive cervical cancers are mainly evident in countries with organized screening programmes.

Annual percentage change in incidence of invasive cervical cancers
1950s–2000
selected Western European countries

organized screening programme initiated at some point during period

no organized screening programme during the period

| Finland | Sweden | France | Switzerland | Denmark | England and Scotland | Netherlands | Italy | Norway | Estonia | Czech Republic |
| 955–99 | 1964–98 | 1978–97 | 1983–97 | 1979–98 | 1978–97 | 1989–98 | 1983–97 | 1953–97 | 1971–2000 | 1985–99 |

-4.7%   -4.2%   -4.2%   -3.7%   -2.4%   -2.3%   -1.6%   -1.4%   -1.1%   -0.6%   -0.6%

1.5%
1968–97
Slovakia

3.5%
1985–99
Slovenia

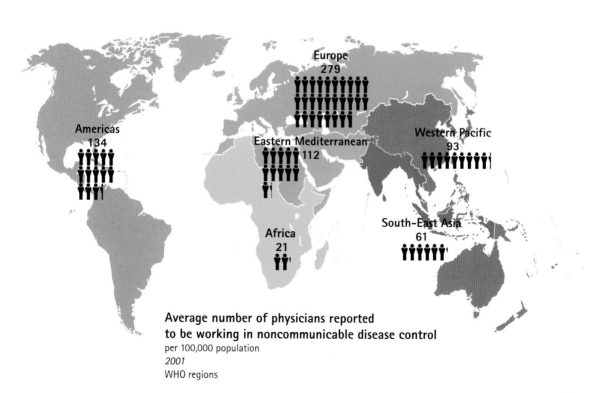

Europe
279

Americas
134

Eastern Mediterranean
112

Western Pacific
93

Africa
21

South-East Asia
61

Average number of physicians reported to be working in noncommunicable disease control
per 100,000 population
2001
WHO regions

"A man too busy to take care of his health is like a mechanic too busy to take care of his tools."
Spanish proverb

Early detection of cancer includes two core components, education and screening. Educational efforts must promote public awareness of the early signs of certain cancers (oral cavity, larynx, colon, rectum, skin, breast, cervix, urinary bladder and prostate) as well as proper follow-up with healthcare providers if these symptoms present. This is particularly important in developing countries, where insufficient resources limit the availability of screening programmes.

The burden of cancer in the population, availability of effective treatment and evidence of benefits and cost-effectiveness, all determine whether screening recommendations become national policies. Most developed and medium-resource countries have programmes and/or national policies for cervical cancer screening (cytology tests) and breast cancer screening (mammography), but few have the same for colorectal cancer screening – faecal occult blood test (FOBT), sigmoidoscopy and colonoscopy. Recommendations for early prostate cancer detection (PSA testing), lung cancer screening (spiral CT) and a low-cost approach towards cervical cancer screening (visual inspection for lesions after applying acetic acid or Lugol's iodine) are pending the results of current investigations.

Early detection can help reduce cancer mortality, yet this depends largely upon proper diagnostic and treatment follow-up, the health service infrastructure of each country and target population compliance.

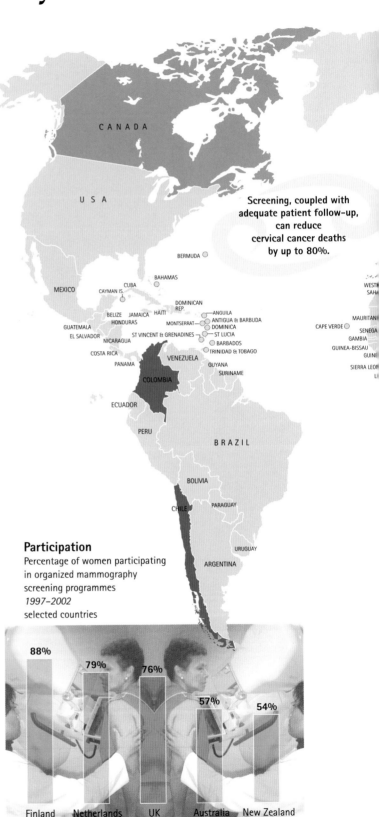

Screening, coupled with adequate patient follow-up, can reduce cervical cancer deaths by up to 80%.

Participation
Percentage of women participating in organized mammography screening programmes
1997–2002
selected countries

88% Finland
79% Netherlands
76% UK
57% Australia
54% New Zealand

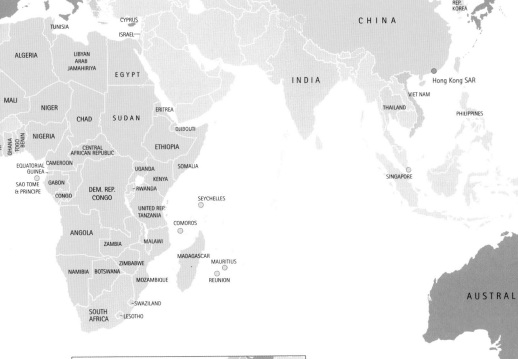

Cervical cancer screening programmes
2004

- national screening programme
- sub-national screening programme
- pilot screening programme
- public health policy only (no population-based screening programme)
- no programme or policy
- no data

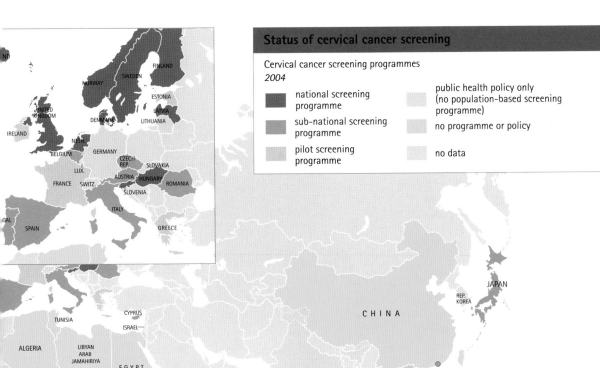

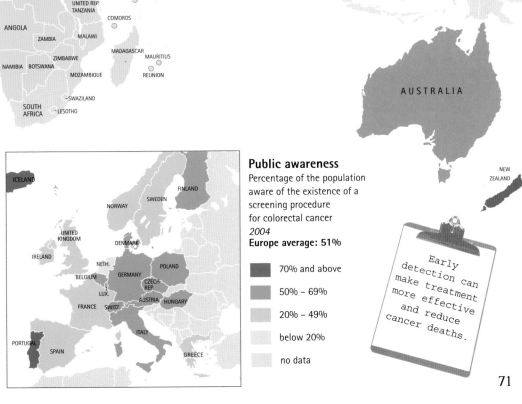

Public awareness

Percentage of the population aware of the existence of a screening procedure for colorectal cancer
2004
Europe average: 51%

- 70% and above
- 50% – 69%
- 20% – 49%
- below 20%
- no data

Early detection can make treatment more effective and reduce cancer deaths.

71

"Men worry over the great number of diseases, while doctors worry over the scarcity of effective remedies."
Bian Que, Chinese physician, c 500 BCE

The diagnosis of cancer is not a death sentence. Advances in treatments – surgery, radiotherapy, chemotherapy – and other forms of medical care for cancer have enhanced survival for many patients. For example, improved forms of chemotherapy have increased the five-year survival rates for children with cancer to greater than 70 percent in northern and western Europe and the USA.

However, the availability of treatment worldwide varies considerably. Radiotherapy, appropriate for treating approximately a half of all cancer patients, is just one example. Developed countries comprise about 15 percent of the world population, yet possess 80 percent of all electron accelerator machines and more than 30 percent of all cobalt machines. Several nations in Africa and Asia lack even one such machine. Other developing nations have very few machines, a situation further complicated by shortages of qualified radiotherapy specialists. Lack of sophisticated technology in these countries often leaves palliative care, which can be provided relatively simply and inexpensively, as the only realistic treatment option.

Problems also exist in developed nations, where the treatment given can vary according to the patient's geographical location, socio-economic status and age. Overall, governmental authorities must focus on assuring equal access to effective treatments for all cancer patients.

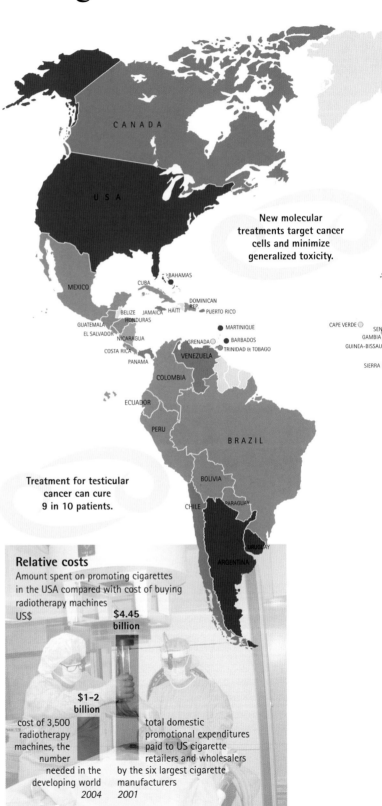

New molecular treatments target cancer cells and minimize generalized toxicity.

Treatment for testicular cancer can cure 9 in 10 patients.

Relative costs
Amount spent on promoting cigarettes in the USA compared with cost of buying radiotherapy machines
US$

$4.45 billion

$1–2 billion

cost of 3,500 radiotherapy machines, the number needed in the developing world
2004

total domestic promotional expenditures paid to US cigarette retailers and wholesalers by the six largest cigarette manufacturers
2001

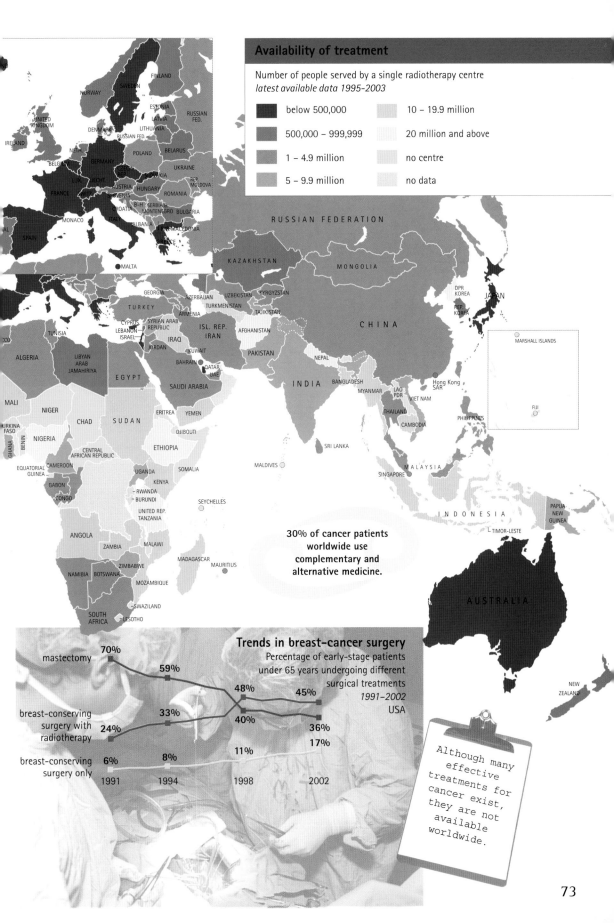

Availability of treatment

Number of people served by a single radiotherapy centre
latest available data 1995-2003

below 500,000	10 – 19.9 million
500,000 – 999,999	20 million and above
1 – 4.9 million	no centre
5 – 9.9 million	no data

30% of cancer patients worldwide use complementary and alternative medicine.

Trends in breast-cancer surgery

Percentage of early-stage patients under 65 years undergoing different surgical treatments
1991-2002
USA

	1991	1994	1998	2002
mastectomy	70%	59%	48%	45%
breast-conserving surgery with radiotherapy	24%	33%	40%	36%
breast-conserving surgery only	6%	8%	11%	17%

Although many effective treatments for cancer exist, they are not available worldwide.

"Strong reasons make strong actions."
William Shakespeare, *King John* III iv, 1596

Cancer organizations are a powerful force in the struggle to ease the burden of cancer. These organizations perform many different functions, but all are dedicated to understanding cancer better, and improving outcomes for cancer patients, cancer survivors, and those touched by cancer. There are numerous other involved partners, including organizations concerned with law, tobacco, nutrition, environment, economic development, women's health, and infectious diseases.

For information about specific cancer organizations worldwide see Useful contacts, page 123. These contacts include members of the International Union Against Cancer (UICC), an international, non-profit association of more than 260 cancer-fighting organizations.

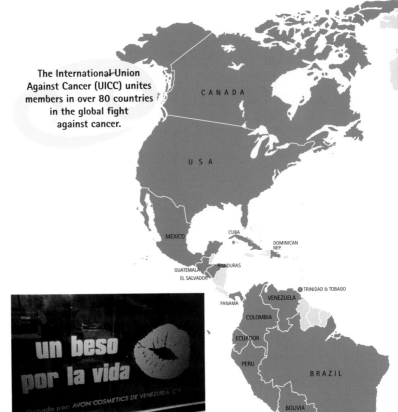

The International Union Against Cancer (UICC) unites members in over 80 countries in the global fight against cancer.

Developing alliances and partnerships: a South American success story

The Venezuela Cancer Society (VCS) has joined forces with Avon Venezuela to set up breast-diagnostic centres in three cities. These centres serve women of all socio-economic backgrounds, and offer diagnostic services not available through the country's public health-care system. Avon provides the funding, and gives VCS autonomy to decide how to use it. VCS has purchased equipment for ultrasonography and stereotactic biopsies, and set up diagnostic centres in established clinics.

UICC World Cancer Congresses

1st	1933	Madrid, Spain
2nd	1936	Brussels, Belgium
3rd	1939	Atlantic City, USA
4th	1947	St. Louis, USA
5th	1950	Paris, France
6th	1954	Sao Paolo, Brazil
7th	1958	London, UK
8th	1962	Moscow, USSR
9th	1966	Tokyo, Japan
10th	1970	Houston, USA
11th	1974	Florence, Italy
12th	1978	Buenos Aires, Argentina
13th	1982	Seattle, USA
14th	1986	Budapest, Hungary
15th	1990	Hamburg, Germany
16th	1994	New Delhi, India
17th	1998	Rio de Janeiro, Brazil
18th	2002	Oslo, Norway
19th	2006	Washington DC, USA

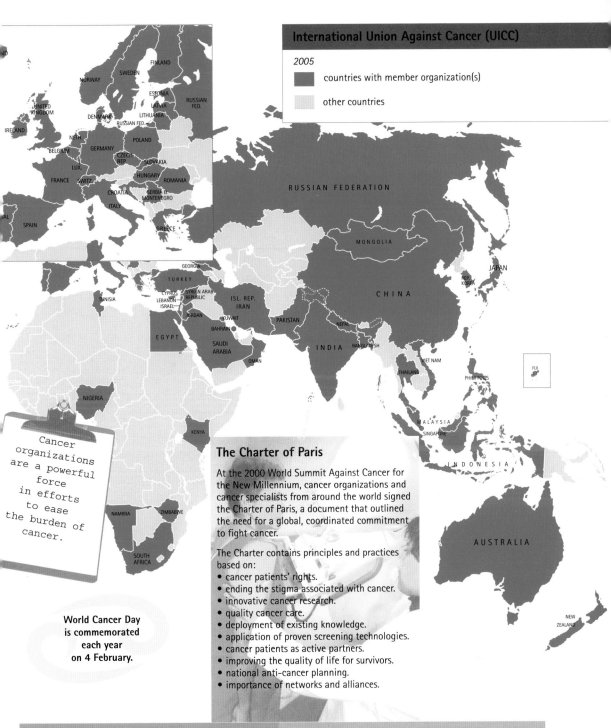

2005

■ countries with member organization(s)

□ other countries

> Cancer organizations are a powerful force in efforts to ease the burden of cancer.

World Cancer Day is commemorated each year on 4 February.

The Charter of Paris

At the 2000 World Summit Against Cancer for the New Millennium, cancer organizations and cancer specialists from around the world signed the Charter of Paris, a document that outlined the need for a global, coordinated commitment to fight cancer.

The Charter contains principles and practices based on:
• cancer patients' rights.
• ending the stigma associated with cancer.
• innovative cancer research.
• quality cancer care.
• deployment of existing knowledge.
• application of proven screening technologies.
• cancer patients as active partners.
• improving the quality of life for survivors.
• national anti-cancer planning.
• importance of networks and alliances.

Types of cancer organizations:

• general, focusing on all aspects of cancer
• specific type of clinical care (i.e. diagnostic, hospice)
• site-specific (i.e., breast, lung)
• focusing on specific population groups (i.e., children, low-income)
• support for patients and survivors
• web-based
• cancer centre, focusing on research and clinical care

Functions of cancer organizations:

• fundraising
• volunteer services
• research
• advocacy
• cancer information
• alliances and partnerships
• health education
• cancer surveillance statistics
• cancer treatment and follow-up
• diagnostic services
• end-of-life care

"The great aim of education is not knowledge but action." Herbert Spencer, British philosopher and sociologist (1820–1903)

While several international days highlight the problem of cancer around the world, many countries also engage in ongoing and sustained campaigns.

Cancer society websites display considerable information on many aspects of cancer. Education directed towards the young emphasizes cancer prevention and a healthy lifestyle. The WHO Global School Health Initiative supports health-promoting schools, with information on deterrents such as a good diet, physical activity and no tobacco use. Educational campaigns for adults advocate changes in lifestyle, such as an improved diet or quitting smoking, and also early detection, such as cervical, breast and colorectal cancer screening. However, much of health education involves one-on-one or small groups.

In 2005, the International Union Against Cancer (UICC) created toolkits for use in cancer campaigns, including logos and slogans suitable for all participating countries, a guide to establishing media partnerships, and campaign materials such as brochures, stickers, posters, press releases and facts sheets.

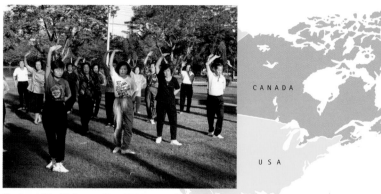

Thailand World Cancer Day 2003

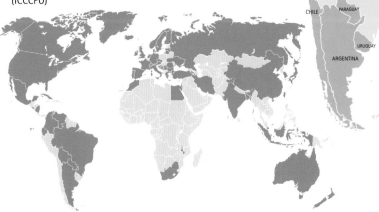

International Childhood Cancer Day 2005
Countries with membership organizations of International Confederation of Childhood Cancer Parent Organizations (ICCCPO)

CANADA

USA

MEXICO

CUBA

BAHAMAS

DOMINICAN REP.

PUERTO RICO

BELIZE JAMAICA HAITI

HONDURAS

ST KITTS & NEVIS

ANTIGUA & BARBUDA

DOMINICA

GUATEMALA

ST VINCENT & GRENADINES

ST LUCIA

EL SALVADOR

NICARAGUA

GRENADA

BARBADOS

TRINIDAD & TOBAGO

COSTA RICA

PANAMA

VENEZUELA

GUYANA

SURINAME

COLOMBIA

FRENCH GUIANA

ECUADOR

PERU

BRAZIL

BOLIVIA

CHILE

PARAGUAY

URUGUAY

ARGENTINA

World cancer days in 2005

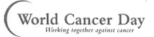

World Cancer Day
4 February

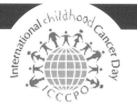

International
Childhood Cancer Day
15 February

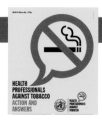

World No Tobacco Day
31 May

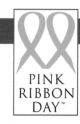

Breast Cancer Pink
Ribbon Day
varies

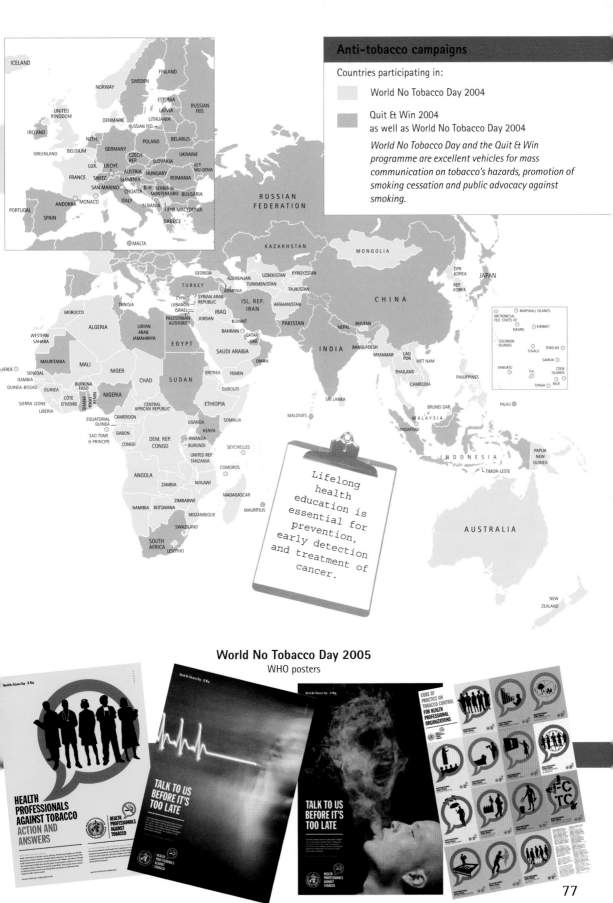

Anti-tobacco campaigns

Countries participating in:

World No Tobacco Day 2004

Quit & Win 2004
as well as World No Tobacco Day 2004

World No Tobacco Day and the Quit & Win programme are excellent vehicles for mass communication on tobacco's hazards, promotion of smoking cessation and public advocacy against smoking.

Lifelong health education is essential for prevention, early detection and treatment of cancer.

World No Tobacco Day 2005
WHO posters

HEALTH PROFESSIONALS AGAINST TOBACCO
ACTION AND ANSWERS

TALK TO US BEFORE IT'S TOO LATE

TALK TO US BEFORE IT'S TOO LATE

CODE OF PRACTICE ON TOBACCO CONTROL FOR HEALTH PROFESSIONAL ORGANIZATIONS

26 | Policies and legislation

> "The people's good is the highest law."
> Cicero (106–43 BCE), *De Legibus*

A WHO survey of 167 countries in all six WHO regions in 2001 assessed national capacity for prevention and control of cancer. Nearly half the countries responding had a cancer control policy or plan. About two-thirds had national guidelines on prevention, and half had guidelines on management. Yet only a few countries had developed nationwide, comprehensive cancer control programmes that included prevention, early detection, treatment and palliative care.

The 2004 WHO Framework Convention on Tobacco Control is the first internationally binding treaty with the aim of reducing non-communicable diseases. Its provisions set international standards on tobacco price and tax increases, tobacco advertising and sponsorship, labelling, illicit trade, second-hand smoke and cessation. It was signed – a non-legally binding intent – by 168 signatories, and came into effect on 27 February 2005, making it one of fastest-track international treaties of all time.

Contracting Parties are bound by international requirement to implement the treaty. The FCTC has already rallied hundreds of non-governmental organizations (NGOs) and encouraged governments to act.

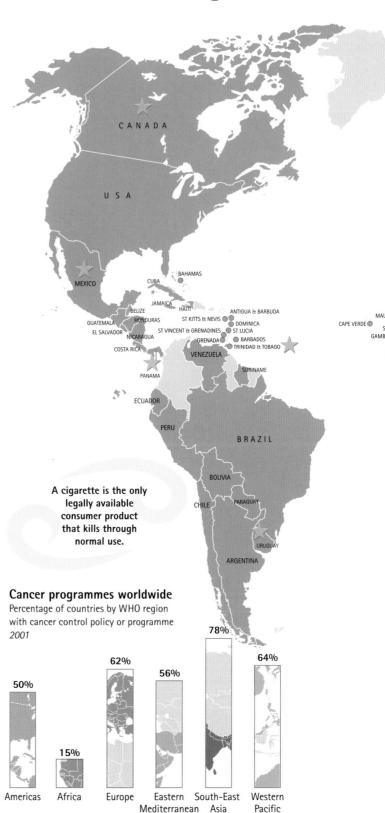

A cigarette is the only legally available consumer product that kills through normal use.

Cancer programmes worldwide
Percentage of countries by WHO region with cancer control policy or programme *2001*

- Americas 50%
- Africa 15%
- Europe 62%
- Eastern Mediterranean 56%
- South-East Asia 78%
- Western Pacific 64%

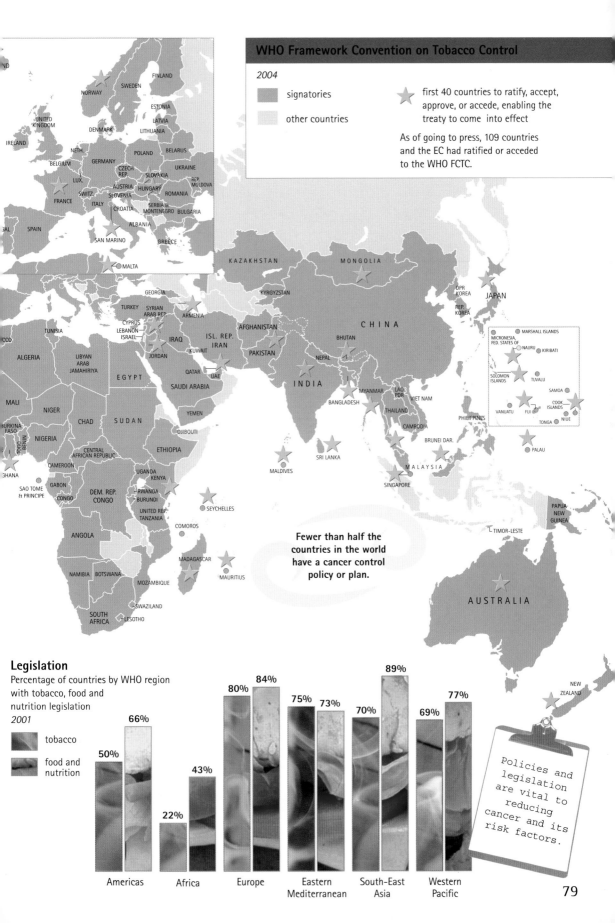

WHO Framework Convention on Tobacco Control

2004

- signatories
- other countries

★ first 40 countries to ratify, accept, approve, or accede, enabling the treaty to come into effect

As of going to press, 109 countries and the EC had ratified or acceded to the WHO FCTC.

Fewer than half the countries in the world have a cancer control policy or plan.

Map labels:

IRELAND, UNITED KINGDOM, NORWAY, SWEDEN, FINLAND, DENMARK, NETH., BELGIUM, LUX., FRANCE, SWITZ., SPAIN, SAN MARINO, ITALY, GERMANY, ESTONIA, LATVIA, LITHUANIA, POLAND, BELARUS, CZECH REP., SLOVAKIA, AUSTRIA, SLOVENIA, HUNGARY, CROATIA, SERBIA & MONTENEGRO, ALBANIA, GREECE, UKRAINE, REP. MOLDOVA, ROMANIA, BULGARIA, MALTA

CCO, ALGERIA, TUNISIA, LIBYAN ARAB JAMAHIRIYA, EGYPT, MALI, NIGER, CHAD, SUDAN, NIGERIA, BURKINA FASO, TOGO, BENIN, GHANA, CAMEROON, CENTRAL AFRICAN REPUBLIC, ETHIOPIA, DJIBOUTI, YEMEN, SAUDI ARABIA, QATAR, UAE, KUWAIT, IRAQ, JORDAN, ISRAEL, LEBANON, CYPRUS, SYRIAN ARAB REP., TURKEY, GEORGIA, ARMENIA, AFGHANISTAN, ISL. REP. IRAN, PAKISTAN, KAZAKHSTAN, KYRGYZSTAN, MONGOLIA, CHINA, DPR KOREA, REP. KOREA, JAPAN, BHUTAN, NEPAL, INDIA, BANGLADESH, MYANMAR, LAO PDR, VIET NAM, THAILAND, CAMBODIA, BRUNEI DAR., MALAYSIA, SINGAPORE, PHILIPPINES, SRI LANKA, MALDIVES, PALAU

SAO TOME & PRINCIPE, GABON, CONGO, DEM. REP. CONGO, UGANDA, KENYA, RWANDA, BURUNDI, UNITED REP. TANZANIA, SEYCHELLES, COMOROS, ANGOLA, NAMIBIA, BOTSWANA, MOZAMBIQUE, MADAGASCAR, MAURITIUS, SWAZILAND, SOUTH AFRICA, LESOTHO

MICRONESIA, FED. STATES OF, MARSHALL ISLANDS, NAURU, KIRIBATI, SOLOMON ISLANDS, TUVALU, SAMOA, VANUATU, FIJI, COOK ISLANDS, TONGA, NIUE

PAPUA NEW GUINEA, TIMOR-LESTE, AUSTRALIA, NEW ZEALAND

Legislation

Percentage of countries by WHO region with tobacco, food and nutrition legislation

2001

- tobacco
- food and nutrition

Region	tobacco	food and nutrition
Americas	50%	66%
Africa	22%	43%
Europe	80%	84%
Eastern Mediterranean	75%	73%
South-East Asia	70%	89%
Western Pacific	69%	77%

Policies and legislation are vital to reducing cancer and its risk factors.

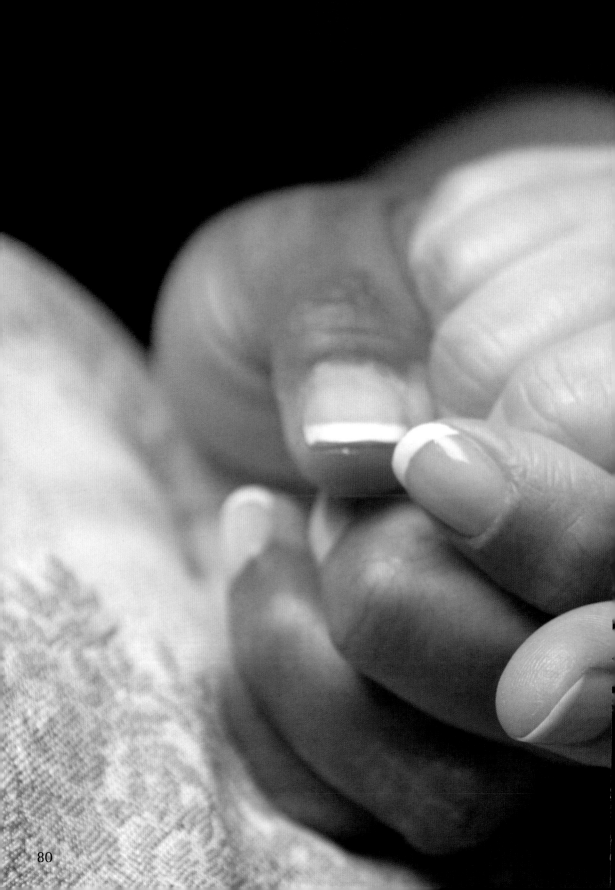

PART SIX

THE FUTURE & THE PAST

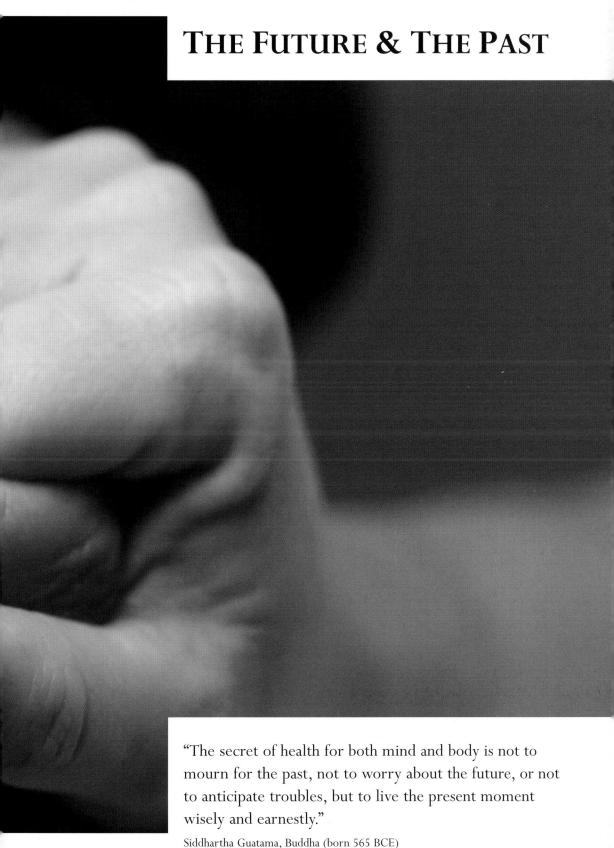

"The secret of health for both mind and body is not to mourn for the past, not to worry about the future, or not to anticipate troubles, but to live the present moment wisely and earnestly."

Siddhartha Guatama, Buddha (born 565 BCE)

> "Let him who would enjoy a good future waste none of his present."
> Roger Ward Babson, American statistician, business forecaster and author (1875–1967)

Predictions are speculative, but some things are certain: the global epidemic of cancer, with its attendant health and economic burden, is not only increasing but is also shifting from developed to developing nations.

The predicted number of new cases of cancer is mostly due to a steadily increasing proportion of elderly people in the world. If current smoking levels and the adoption of unhealthy lifestyles persist, the increase will be even greater.

By 2020, cancer could kill more than 10 million people a year. If action is taken now, 2 million lives can be saved each per year by 2020, and 6.5 million by 2040.

No matter what advances there may be in high-technology medicine, any major reduction in deaths and disability from cancer will come from prevention, not from cure.

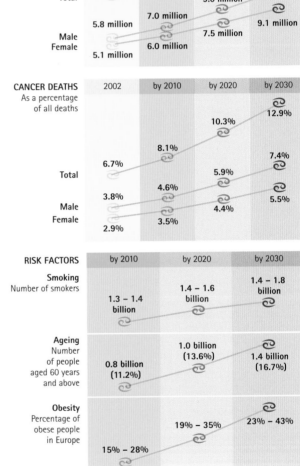

NEW CANCER CASES
Annual number

	2002	by 2010	by 2020	by 2030
Total	10.9 million	13.0 million	16.5 million	20.3 million
Male	5.8 million	7.0 million	9.0 million	11.2 million
Female	5.1 million	6.0 million	7.5 million	9.1 million

CANCER DEATHS
As a percentage of all deaths

	2002	by 2010	by 2020	by 2030
Total	6.7%	8.1%	10.3%	12.9%
Male	3.8%	4.6%	5.9%	7.4%
Female	2.9%	3.5%	4.4%	5.5%

RISK FACTORS

	by 2010	by 2020	by 2030
Smoking — Number of smokers	1.3 – 1.4 billion	1.4 – 1.6 billion	1.4 – 1.8 billion
Ageing — Number of people aged 60 years and above	0.8 billion (11.2%)	1.0 billion (13.6%)	1.4 billion (16.7%)
Obesity — Percentage of obese people in Europe	15% – 28%	19% – 35%	23% – 43%

New cancer cases

Number, excluding skin cancer, by WHO region *2002 and 2020 projected* thousands

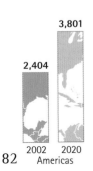
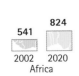
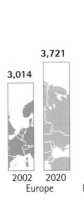
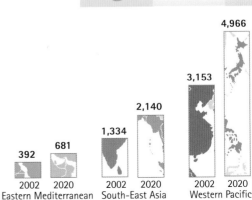

	2002	2020
Americas	2,404	3,801
Africa	541	824
Europe	3,014	3,721
Eastern Mediterranean	392	681
South-East Asia	1,334	2,140
Western Pacific	3,153	4,966

ACTION	by 2010	by 2020	by 2030
Prevention	Anti-viral vaccines, currently available for hepatitis B, developed for the papilloma virus which causes cervical cancer. More drugs developed that will prevent cancer and/or the development of chemo-prevention programmes for the treatment of high-risk individuals for some cancers.	Anti-viral vaccines developed for other viruses which cause cancer. Treatment will target specific cancer cells and not affect the body's healthy cells.	Therapeutic vaccines linked to personal genetic profiles.
Research and development	New causes of cancer discovered, including bacteria, viruses, chemicals and pollution. Better understanding of the role of food and nutrition in cancer.	Self-stem cells (cells taken from patient's body) used to grow new tissues after surgery.	Bio-engineered tissues available for replacement tissues.

	by 2010	by 2020	by 2030
UN Conventions and Goals	WHO Framework Convention on Tobacco Control (FCTC) ratified by all countries. WHO Global Strategy on Cancer implemented by most countries.	WHO convention on food (covering content, labelling, taxation, advertising) ratified. Millennium Development Goals (2015): As cancer and other non-communicable diseases cause poverty, access to affordable essential drugs in developing countries provided, in cooperation with pharmaceutical companies.	Convention on universal access to essential preventive healthcare and equity in its quality and delivery.

> Any major reduction in cancer deaths will come from prevention, not cure.

	by 2010	by 2020	by 2030
Miscellaneous treatment	Personal medical records stored on smart card. Vaccine to boost immune system reduces relapses in people who have had cancer.	Health systems driven by primary health care to ensure universal access to quality health care services. Instantaneous language translation software enables patients to be understood by health professionals in any country.	In developed countries, patients' knowledge of their own health may equal that of their doctors in the 1990s. Cancer will be seen as a chronic disease like high-blood pressure or diabetes. Patients co-exist with their cancers as long as they take their medications.
Diagnosis and investigations	X-rays, Magnetic Resonance Imaging (MRI) and ultrasound images transmitted electronically to diagnostic centre (which may be abroad).	A minuscule computer, with micro-sensors automatically sensing and recording health data, could be part of everyday wear. Blood tests will be widely available to screen patients for cancer.	
Genetics	More cancer genes identified.	Genetic manipulation to prevent and treat cancer.	Genetic profiling will foresee the cancer risk of each individual patient, raising issues of employment, marriage, insurance, and confidentiality of information. Genetic profiling of cancer tissue predicts how individual cancers will behave and their resistance to treatment, and therefore helps choose the best drug.
Artificial body parts developed		Lungs, liver	
Transplant surgery		Xeno-transplantation with pig body parts soars as rejection problem overcome.	Pig-napping of personal transgenic pigs a new crime.
High technology		Nano-surgeons, or sub-microscopic robots, crawl around the body, targeting and eliminating cancer cells. All newborn babies given CD-ROM containing their unique genomic maps and data with summaries of cancer and other diseases for which they may be at increased risk.	Computerized "auto-doc" machine externally detects and treats cancer by MRI.
Drugs	More tumour-specific and enzyme-blocker drugs developed with very few side effects. Cancer drugs mainly taken by mouth.	Molecular-targeted drugs become routine therapy for some cancers.	"Trial and error" in drug prescription abandoned in favour of personalized prescription.

83

70–80 million years ago
Evidence of cancer cells in dinosaur fossils, found in 2003.

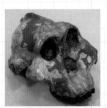

4.2–3.9 million years ago The oldest known hominid malignant tumour was found in Homo erectus or Australopithecus by Louis Leakey in 1932.

3000 BCE *Egypt* Evidence of cancerous cells in mummies.

1900–1600 BCE Cancer found in remains of Bronze Age human female skull.

1750 BCE Babylonian code of Hammurabi set standard fee for surgical removal of tumours (ten shekels) and penalties for failure.

1600 BCE *Egypt* The Egyptians blamed cancers on the Gods. Ancient Egyptian scrolls describe eight cases of breast tumours treated by cauterization.
Stomach cancer treated with boiled barley mixed with dates; cancer of the uterus by a concoction of fresh dates mixed with pig's brain introduced into vagina.

1100–400 BCE *China* Physicians specializing in treating swellings and ulcerations are referred to in *The Rites of the Zhou Dynasty*.

500 BCE *India* Indian epic tale, the Ramayana, describes treatment with arsenic paste to thwart tumour growth.

400 BCE *Peru* Pre-Columbian Inca mummies contain lesions suggestive of malignant melanoma.

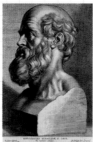

400 BCE
Greece Greek physician Hippocrates (460–370 BCE), the "Father of Medicine", believed illness was caused by imbalance of four bodily humours: yellow bile, black bile, blood, and phlegm. He was the first to recognize differences between benign and malignant tumours.

circa 250 BCE *China* The first clinical picture of breast cancer, including progression, metastasis and death, and prognosis approximately ten years after diagnosis, was described in *The Nei Ching*, or *The Yellow Emperor's Classic of Internal Medicine*. It gave the first description of tumours and five forms of therapy: spiritual, pharmacological, diet, acupuncture, and treatment of respiratory diseases.

50 AD *Italy* The Romans found some tumours could be removed by surgery and cauterized, but thought medicine did not work. They noted some tumours grew again.

100 AD *Italy* Greek doctor Claudius Galen (129–216 AD) removed some tumours surgically, but he generally believed that cancer was best left untreated. Galen believed melancholia the chief factor in causing breast cancer, and recommended special diets, exorcism and topical applications.

500–1500 *Europe* Surgery and cautery were used on smaller tumours. Caustic pastes, usually containing arsenic, were used on more extensive cancers, as well as phlebotomy (blood-letting), diet, herbal medicines, powder of crab and symbolic charms.

1400–1500s *Italy* Leonardo da Vinci (1452–1519) dissected cadavers for artistic and scientific purposes, adding to the knowledge of the human body.

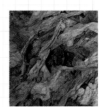

1492 Christopher Columbus returned to Europe from the Americas with the first tobacco leaves and seeds ever seen on the continent. A crew member, Rodrigo de Jerez, was seen smoking and imprisoned by the Inquisition, which believed he was possessed by the devil.

1500 *Europe* Autopsies were conducted more often and understanding of internal cancers grew.

1595 *Netherlands* Zacharias Janssen invented the first compound microscope.

17th century *Netherlands* Dutch surgeon Adrian Helvetius performed both lumpectomy and mastectomy, claiming this cured breast cancer.

17th century *Germany* Cancer surgery techniques improved, but lack of anaesthesia and antiseptic conditions made surgery a risky choice. German surgeon Wilhelm Fabricius Hildanus (1560–1634), removed enlarged lymph nodes in breast cancer operations, while Johann Scultetus (1595–1645) performed total mastectomies.

17th century *France* Physician Claude Gendron (1663–1750) concluded that cancer arises locally as a hard, growing mass, untreatable with drugs, and that it must be removed with all its "filaments".

17th century *Netherlands* Professor Hermann Boerhaave (1668–1738) believed inflammation could result in cancer.

17th–18th centuries *Netherlands* Antony van Leeuwenhoek (1632–1723) refined the single lens microscope and was the first to see blood cells and bacteria, aiding the better understanding of cells, blood and lymphatic system – major steps in improving the understanding of cancer.

France Physician Le Dran (1685–1770) first recognized that breast cancer could spread to the regional auxiliary lymph nodes, carrying a poorer prognosis.

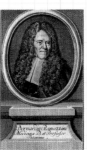

1700 *Italy* Dr Bernardino Ramazzini (1633–1714), a founder of occupational/industrial medicine, reported the virtual absence of cervical cancer and relatively high incidence of breast cancer in nuns. This observation was an important step toward identifying hormonal factors such as pregnancy and infections related to sexual contact in cancer risk, and was the first indication that lifestyle might affect the development of cancer.

1733–88 *France* Physicians and scientists performed systematic experiments on cancer, leading to oncology as a medical specialty. Two French scientists – physician Jean

Astruc and chemist Bernard Peyrilhe – were key to these new investigations.

1761 *Padua, Italy* Giovanni Morgagni performed the first autopsies to relate the patient's illness to the science of disease, laying the foundation for modern pathology.

1761 *UK* Dr John Hill published "Cautions Against the Immoderate Use of Snuff", the first report linking tobacco and cancer.

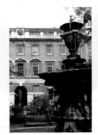

1775 *UK* Dr Percival Pott of Saint Bartholomew's Hospital in London described cancer in chimney sweeps caused by soot collecting under their scrotum, the first indication that exposure to chemicals in the environment could cause cancer. This research led to many additional studies that identified other occupational carcinogens and thence to public health measures to reduce cancer risk.

1779 *France* First cancer hospital founded in Reims. It was forced to move from the city because people believed cancer was contagious.

18th century *Scotland* Scottish surgeon John Hunter (1728–93) stated that tumours originated in the lymph system and then seeded around the body. He suggested that some cancers might be cured by surgery, especially those that had not invaded nearby tissue.

19th century *Scotland* In the early 1800s, Scottish physician John Waldrop proposed that "glioma of the retina", which typically appeared within the eyes of

new-borns and young children and was usually lethal, might be cured via early removal of affected organs.

1829 *France* Gynaecologist Joseph Recamier described the invasion of the bloodstream by cancer cells, coining the term metastasis, which came to mean the distant spread of cancer from its primary site to other places in the body.

1838 *Germany* Pathologist Johannes Müller demonstrated that cancer is made up of cells and not lymph. His student, Rudolph Virchow (1821–1902), later proposed that chronic inflammation – the site of a wound that never heals – was the cause of cancer.

1842 *Italy* Domenico Antonio Rigoni-Stern undertook first major statistical analysis of cancer incidence and mortality using 1760–1839 data from Verona. This showed that more women than men died from tumours, and that the commonest female cancers were breast and uterine (each accounting for a third of total deaths). He found cancer death rates for both sexes were rising and concluded that incidence of cancer increases with age, that cancer is found less in the country than in the city, and that unmarried people are more likely to contract the disease.

1845 *Scotland* John Hughes Bennett, 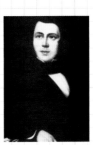 the Edinburgh physician, was the first to describe leukaemia as an excessive proliferation of blood cells.

1851–1971 *UK* Decennial reports linked cancer death to occupation and social class.

1880–1956

1880 Earlier invention of general anaesthesia (chloroform, ether, nitrous oxide) became more widespread, making cancer surgery more acceptable.

1881 *USA* First practical cigarette-making machine patented by James Bonsack. It could produce 120,000 cigarettes a day, each machine doing the work of 48 people. Production costs plummeted, and – with the invention of the safety match a few decades later – cigarette-smoking began its explosive growth.

1886 *Brazil* Hereditary basis for cancer first suggested after Professor Hilario de Gouvea of the Medical School in Rio de Janeiro reported a family with increased susceptibility to retinoblastoma.

1890s *USA* Professor William Stewart Halsted at Johns Hopkins University developed the radical mastectomy for breast cancer, removing breast, underlying muscles and lymph nodes under the arm.

1895 *Germany* Physicist Wilhelm Konrad Roentgen (1845–1923) discovered X-rays, used in the diagnosis of cancer. Within a few years this led to the use of radiation for cancer treatment.

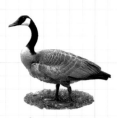

1897 *USA* Walter B Cannon (1871–1945) was still a college student when he fed bismuth and barium mixtures to geese, outlining their gullets on an X-ray plate (the fore-runner of the Barium meal examination).

19th century Invention and use of the modern microscope, which later helped identify cancer cells.

19th century *Germany* Johannes Müller's student Rudolph Virchow (1821–1902), "the founder of cellular pathology", determined that all cells, including cancer cells, are derived from other cells. He was the first to coin the term "leukaemia" and believed chronic inflammation was the cause of cancer.

19th century *Germany* Surgeon Karl Thiersch showed cancers metastasize through the spread of malignant cells.

1800s *UK* Surgeon Stephen Paget (1855–1926) first deduced that cancer cells spread to all organs of the body by the bloodstream, but only grow in the organ ("soil") they find compatible. This laid the groundwork for the true understanding of metastasis.

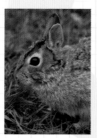

1895 *Scotland* Dr Thomas Beatson discovered that the breasts of rabbits stopped producing milk after he removed the ovaries. This control of one organ over another led Beatson to test what would happen if the ovaries were removed in patients suffering from advanced breast cancer, and he found that oophorectomy often resulted in improvement. He thus discovered the stimulating effect of oestrogen on breast tumours long before the hormone was discovered. This work provided a foundation for the modern use of hormones and analogues (eg tamoxifen, taxol) for treatment and prevention of breast cancer.

before 1900 Lung cancer was extremely rare; now it is one of the commonest cancers.

by 1900 Hundreds of materials, both man-made and natural, were recognized as causes of cancer (carcinogens).

1902 X-ray exposure led to skin cancer on the hand of a lab technician. Within a decade, many more physicians and scientists, unaware of the dangers of radiation, developed a variety of cancers.

1905 *UK* Physicians at the Royal Ophthalmology Hospital reported the first case of "hereditary" retinal glioma, which presented in the child of a parent cured of the disease.

1907 *USA* Epidemiological study found that meat-eating Germans, Irish, and Scandinavians living in Chicago had higher rates of cancer than did Italians and Chinese, who ate considerably less meat.

1910 *Austria* First national cancer society founded: Austrian Cancer Society.

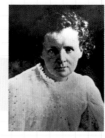

1911 *France* Marie Curie was awarded a second Nobel Prize, this time in Chemistry, in recognition of her work in radioactivity.

1900–1950 Radiotherapy – the use of radiation to kill cancer cells or stop them dividing – was developed as a treatment.

1911 *USA* Peyton Rous (1879–1970) proved that viruses caused cancer in chickens, for which he was eventually awarded the Nobel Prize in 1966.

1913 *USA* The American Cancer Society was founded as the American Society for the Control of Cancer (ASCC) by 15 physicians and business leaders in New York City. In 1945 the ASCC was renamed the American Cancer Society. It remains the world's largest voluntary organization.

1915 *Japan* Cancer was induced in laboratory animals for the first time by a chemical, coal tar, applied to rabbits' skin at Tokyo University. Soon many other substances were observed to be carcinogens, including benzene, hydrocarbons, aniline, asbestos and tobacco.

1928 *Greece, USA* George Papanicolaou (1883–1962) identified malignant cells among the normal cast off vaginal cells of women with cancer of the cervix, which led to the Pap smear test.

1930 *Germany* Researchers in Cologne drew the first statistical connection between smoking and cancer.

1930s *Puerto Rico* Dr Cornelius Rhoads, a pathologist, allegedly injected his Puerto Rican subjects with cancer cells – 13 people died.

1933 International Union Against Cancer (UICC) founded.

1933 *Spain* First World Cancer Congress held in Madrid.

1930s–1950s Classification of breast cancer introduced, enabling the planning of more rational treatment tailored to the individual.

1934 *UK* Wood and Gloyne reported first two cases of lung cancer linked to asbestos.

1937 *USA* National Cancer Institute inaugurated.

1939 *USA* Drs Alton Ochsner and Michael DeBakey first reported the association of smoking and lung cancer.

1939–45 During the Second World War US Army discovered that nitrogen mustard was effective in treating cancer of the lymph nodes (lymphoma). This was the birth of chemotherapy – the use of drugs to treat cancer.

1943–45 *Denmark, UK* First national cancer registries established.

1947 *Canada* Dr Norman Delarue compared 50 patients with lung cancer with 50 patients hospitalized with other diseases. He discovered that over 90% of the first group – but only half of the second – were smokers, and confidently predicted that by 1950 no one would be smoking.

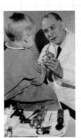

1947 *USA* Sidney Farber (1903–73), one of the founders of the speciality of paediatric pathology, used a derivative of folic acid, methotrexate, to inhibit acute leukaemia in children.

1940s–1950s *USA* Dr Charles B Huggins' (1901–97) research on prostate cancer changed the way scientists regarded the behaviour of all cancer cells, and for the first time brought hope to the prospect of treating advanced cancers. He showed that cancer cells were not autonomous and self-perpetuating but were dependent on chemical signals such as hormones to grow and survive, and that depriving

cancer cells of these signals could restore the health of patients with widespread metastases. He was awarded the Nobel Prize in 1966 (shared with Peyton Rous).

1950 *USA* Gertrude Elion (1918–99) created a purine chemical, which she developed into 6-mercaptopurine, or 6-MP. It was rapidly approved for use in childhood leukaemia. She received the Nobel Prize in 1988.

1950 *USA* The link between smoking and lung cancer was confirmed. A landmark article from *The Journal of the American Medical Association* appeared on 27 May 1950: "Tobacco smoking as a possible etiologic factor in bronchogenic carcinoma" by E L Wynder and Evarts Graham. The same issue featured a full-page ad for Chesterfields with the actress Gene Tierney and golfer Ben Hogan; the journal accepted tobacco ads until 1953.

1951 *UK* Dr Richard Doll and Prof Austin Bradford Hill conducted first large-scale study of link between smoking and lung cancer.

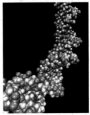

1953 *UK* James Watson and Francis Crick described the double helical structure of DNA, marking the beginning of the modern era of genetics.

1954 *USA* First tobacco litigation against the cigarette companies, brought by a widow on behalf of her smoker husband, who died from cancer. The cigarette companies won.

1956 *USA* Dr Min Chiu Li (–1980) first demonstrated clinically that chemotherapy could result in the cure of a widely metastatic malignant disease.

1960–2005

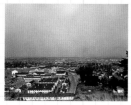

1960 *Japan* Group cancer screening for stomach cancer began with a mobile clinic in Tohoku region.

1960 *USA* Dr Min Chiu Li published another important and original finding: the use of multiple-agent combination chemotherapy for the treatment of metastatic cancers of the testis. Twenty years later, it was demonstrated that combination chemotherapy, combined with techniques for local control, had virtually eliminated deaths from testicular malignancy.

1963 *Japan* Cancer research programmes were established by the Ministry of Health and Welfare and the Ministry of Education, Science and Culture.

1964 *USA* First US Surgeon General's report on smoking and health.

1965 WHO established International Agency for Research on Cancer (IARC) based in Lyons, France.

1966 International Association of Cancer Registries (IACR) founded.

1960s–1970s Trials in several countries demonstrated the effectiveness of mammography screening for breast cancer.

1970s *USA, Italy* Bernard Fisher in the USA and Umberto Veronesi in Italy both launched long-term studies as to whether lumpectomy followed by radiation therapy was an option to radical mastectomy in early breast cancer. These studies concluded that total mastectomy offered no advantage over either lumpectomy or lumpectomy plus radiation therapy.

1971 *USA* The National Cancer Act in President Nixon's "War on Cancer" mandated financial support for cancer research, established a network of population-based cancer registries, outlined intervention strategies and, in 1973 established the SEER (Surveillance, Epidemiology and End Results).

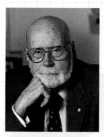

1973 *USA* Bone marrow transplantation first performed successfully on a dog in Seattle by Dr E Donnall Thomas (1920–). This led to human bone marrow transplantation, resulting in cures for leukaemias and lymphomas. In 1990 Dr Thomas won a Nobel Prize for his work.

1970s Childhood leukaemia became one of the first cancers that could be cured by a combination of drugs.

1970s *USA* Discovery of the first cancer gene (the oncogene, which in certain circumstances can transform a cell into a tumour cell).

1970s onwards WHO, UICC and others promoted national cancer planning for nations to prioritize and focus their cancer activities.

1981 *Japan* Professor Takeshi Hirayama (1923–95) published the first report linking passive smoking and lung cancer in the non-smoking wives of men who smoked.

1981 *Italy* Dr G Bonnadona in Milan performed first study of adjuvant chemotherapy for breast cancer using cyclophosphamide, methotrexate and 5-fluorouracil, resulting in reduction of cancer relapse. Adjuvant chemotherapy is now standard treatment for lung, breast, colon, stomach and ovary cancers.

1980s *USA* Kaposi's sarcoma and T-cell lymphoma linked to AIDs.

1982 *USA* Nobel Laureate Baruch S Blumberg was instrumental in developing a reliable and safe vaccine against hepatitis B (which causes primary liver cancer).

1980s *Australia* Barry Marshall and J Robin Warren identified bacterium h pylori, noting it caused duodenal and gastric ulcers and increased the risks of gastric cancer. H pylori infection can be eradicated with antibiotics. They received the 2005 Nobel Prize for Medicine.

1980s *USA* Vincent DeVita developed a four-drug combination to raise the cure rate of Hodgkin's disease from nearly hopeless to 80%.

mid-1980s Human Genome Project was initiated to pinpoint location 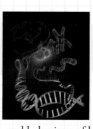 and function of estimated 50,000–100,000 genes that make up the inherited set of "instructions" for functions and behaviour of human beings.

1980s WHO Programme on Cancer Control established.

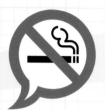

1988 Global First WHO World No Tobacco Day, subsequently an annual event.

1989 European Network of Cancer Registries (ENCR) established.

1989 *USA* National Institutes of Health researchers performed the first approved gene therapy, inserting foreign genes to track tumour-killing cells in cancer patients. This project proved the safety of gene therapy.

1990 *USA* The Breast and Cervical Cancer Mortality Prevention Act signed into US law. Established the only nationwide organized cancer-screening programme in the US, the National Breast and Cervical Cancer Early Detection Programme.

1991 Evidence linking specific environmental carcinogens to telltale DNA damage emerged, eg sun radiation was found to produce change in tumour suppressor genes in skin cells, aflatoxin (a fungus poison) or hepatitis B virus to cause a mutation in the liver, and chemicals in cigarette smoke to switch on a gene that makes lung cells vulnerable to the chemicals' cancer-causing properties.

1994 *USA, Canada, UK, France, Japan* Scientists collaborated and discovered BRCA1, the first breast and ovarian cancer predisposing gene.

1994 *USA* National Programme of Cancer Registries (NPCR) established.

1995 Gene therapy, immune system modulation and genetically engineered antibodies used to treat cancer.

1999 *Netherlands, USA* Jan Walboomers of the Free University of Amsterdam and Michele Manos of Johns Hopkins provided evidence that the human papilloma virus is present in 99.7% of all cases of cervical cancer.

1999 The Bill & Melinda Gates Foundation awarded a five-year, $50 million grant to the Alliance for Cervical Cancer Prevention (ACCP), a group of five international organizations with a shared goal of working to prevent cervical cancer in developing countries.

1999 *France* American Lance Armstrong became an inspiration to cancer survivors around the world when he overcame testicular cancer and won his first of a record seven Tour de France cycling victories.

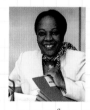

2000 53rd World Health Assembly presided over by Dr Libertina Amathila (Namibia) endorsed "Global strategy for non-communicable disease (NCD) prevention and control", which outlined major objectives for monitoring, preventing and managing NCDs, with special emphasis on major NCDs with common risk factors and determinants – cardiovascular disease, cancer, diabetes and chronic respiratory disease.

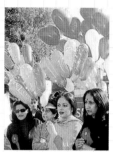

2000 The entire human genome is mapped.

2000 Charter of Paris against Cancer signed.

2001 *Luxembourg* International Childhood Cancer Day was launched, its aim to raise awareness of the 250,000 children worldwide who get cancer every year. Some 80% of these children have little or no access to treatment. The first annual event in 2002 was supported in 30 countries around the world and raised over US$100,000 for parent organizations to help children in their own countries.

2002 *US Cancer Statistics* first published. Provided cancer incidence data covering 78% of US population.

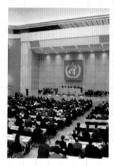

2004 *Geneva, Switzerland* WHO cancer prevention and control resolution approved by World Health Assembly.

2005 WHO Framework Convention on Tobacco Control came into force, using international law to further public health and prevent cancer.

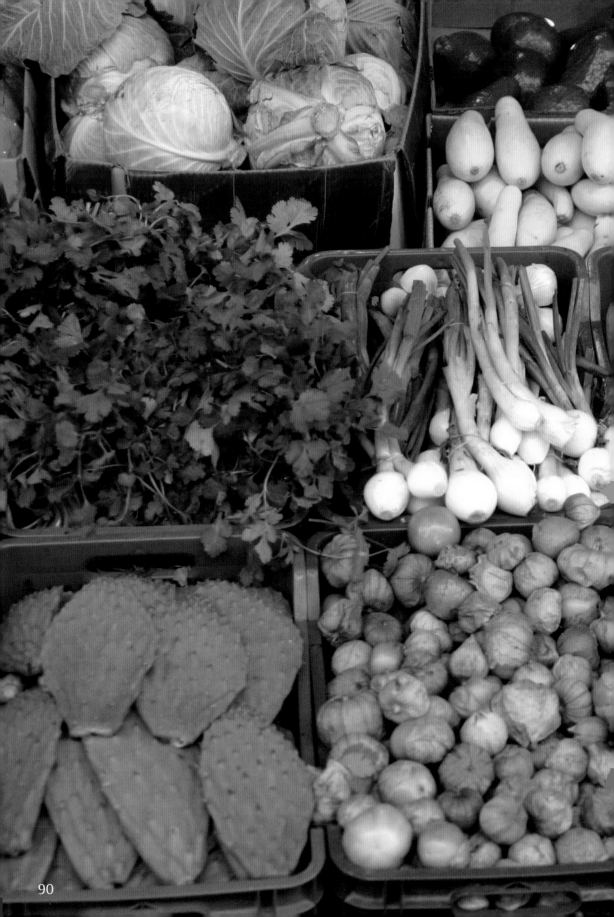

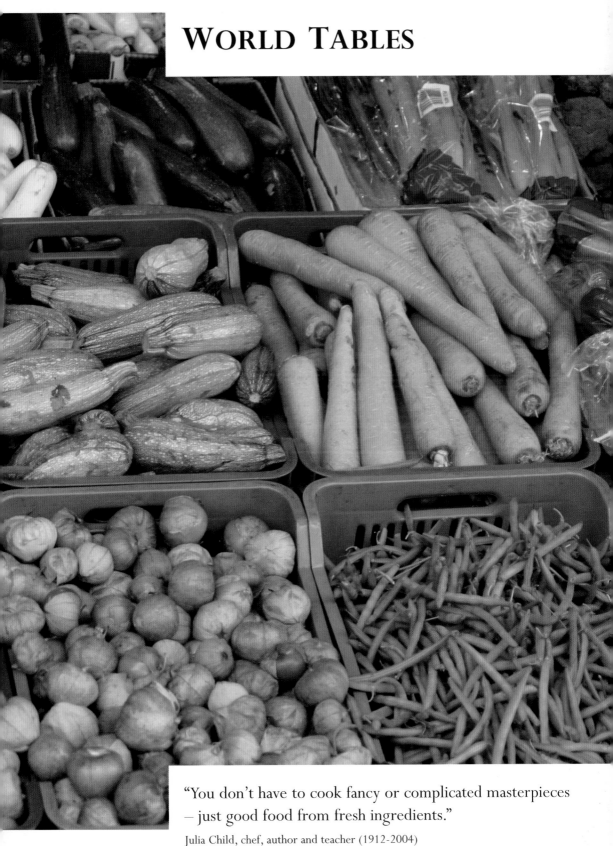

PART SEVEN

WORLD TABLES

"You don't have to cook fancy or complicated masterpieces – just good food from fresh ingredients."

Julia Child, chef, author and teacher (1912-2004)

Table A **Risk factors for cancer**

Countries	1 Population thousands	2 Youth smoking prevalence percentages (national data)	
		male	female
Afghanistan	20,988	–	–
Albania	3,169	9.0%	3.2%
Algeria	31,833	–	–
Angola	13,522	–	–
Antigua and Barbuda	79	0.0%	1.1%
Argentina	36,772	16.4%	28.3%
Armenia	3,056	–	–
Australia	19,881	24.0%	23.0%
Austria	8,090	26.1%	37.1%
Azerbaijan	8,233	–	–
Bahrain	712	11.8%	3.0%
Bangladesh	138,066	–	–
Barbados	271	3.6%	3.6%
Belarus	9,881	36.2%	27.8%
Belgium	10,376		
Belize	274	11.4%	5.9%
Benin	6,720	–	–
Bhutan	874		
Bolivia	8,814	–	–
Bosnia and Herzegovina	4,140	12.8%	5.4%
Botswana	1,722	3.2%	2.3%
Brazil	176,596	–	–
Brunei Darussalam	356	–	–
Bulgaria	7,823	31.2%	35.5%
Burkina Faso	12,109	–	–
Burundi	7,206	–	–
Cambodia	13,404	2.4%	0.0%
Cameroon	16,087	–	–
Canada	31,630	15.5%	13.5%
Cape Verde	470	–	–
Central African Rep.	3,881	–	–
Chad	8,582	–	–
Chile	15,774	–	–
China	1,288,400	–	–
Colombia	44,584	–	–
Comoros	600	–	–
Congo	3,757	–	–
Congo, Dem. Rep.	53,153	–	–
Cook Islands	18	24.7%	24.3%
Costa Rica	4,005	–	–
Côte d'Ivoire	16,835	–	–
Croatia	4,445	23.2%	24.9%
Cuba	11,326	–	–
Cyprus	770	–	–
Czech Republic	10,202	28.7%	30.6%
Denmark	5,387	16.7%	21.0%
Djibouti	705	8.2%	0.0%
Dominica	71	7.0%	4.3%

3 Adult smoking prevalence				4 Overweight prevalence		Countries
percentages			Age span	percentages		
total	male	female	years	male	female	
49.5%	82.0%	17.0%	–	11.2%	15.6%	Afghanistan
39.0%	60.0%	18.0%	15+	57.2%	52.5%	Albania
12.8%	32.3%	0.4%	25–64	32.1%	43.2%	Algeria
–	–	–	–	19.9%	31.4%	Angola
–	–	–	–	50.0%	58.3%	Antigua and Barbuda
28.5%	32.3%	24.9%	18–64	70.1%	62.1%	Argentina
32.1%	61.8%	2.4%	18+	53.9%	52.8%	Armenia
17.4%	18.6%	16.3%	18+	69.7%	60.2%	Australia
29.1%	33.9%	24.2%	25–64	59.0%	53.4%	Austria
–	–	0.6%	–	57.4%	56.8%	Azerbaijan
10.2%	15.0%	3.1%	15+	60.9%	66.0%	Bahrain
40.8%	54.8%	26.7%	18+	5.9%	4.3%	Bangladesh
8.5%	20.1%	0.8%	25+	55.5%	77.8%	Barbados
27.3%	53.2%	7.1%	–	63.7%	69.9%	Belarus
27.0%	30.0%	25.0%	–	49.0%	40.7%	Belgium
–	–	–	–	43.3%	53.3%	Belize
37.0%	–	–	–	15.8%	32.8%	Benin
–	–	–	–	34.0%	44.7%	Bhutan
26.8%	37.6%	19.4%	25+	52.5%	64.4%	Bolivia
37.6%	49.2%	29.7%	18–65	56.6%	51.0%	Bosnia and Herzegovina
21.0%	–	–	–	35.5%	46.9%	Botswana
–	21.8%	14.0%	18+	43.4%	49.2%	Brazil
20.0%	–	–	–	55.3%	61.9%	Brunei Darussalam
32.7%	43.8%	23.0%	16+	62.8%	45.5%	Bulgaria
12.6%	17.7%	0.6%	11–25	10.6%	15.8%	Burkina Faso
14.6%	15.6%	11.4%	19+	7.0%	16.3%	Burundi
35.0%	66.7%	10.0%	15+	9.6%	7.1%	Cambodia
35.7%	–	–	–	35.7%	38.3%	Cameroon
20.0%	22.0%	17.0%	15+	64.5%	55.9%	Canada
–	–	–	–	30.5%	41.8%	Cape Verde
–	–	–	–	6.7%	17.7%	Central African Rep.
–	24.1%	–	–	10.4%	17.1%	Chad
42.4%	48.3%	36.8%	17+	58.9%	64.4%	Chile
–	67.0%	1.9%	18+	27.5%	22.7%	China
18.9%	26.8%	11.3%	18–69	52.7%	55.1%	Colombia
–	–	–	–	17.7%	33.1%	Comoros
7.8%	–	–	–	12.0%	24.2%	Congo
–	–	–	–	4.3%	11.9%	Congo, Dem. Rep.
56.8%	34.4%	71.1%	15+	92.0%	88.5%	Cook Islands
19.4%	29.0%	9.7%	20–49	49.8%	56.2%	Costa Rica
24.4%	42.3%	1.8%	15+	10.9%	32.5%	Côte d'Ivoire
30.3%	34.1%	26.6%	18–65	60.0%	45.3%	Croatia
36.8%	48.1%	26.2%	15+	55.2%	57.0%	Cuba
37.4%	38.5%	7.6%	15+	50.4%	59.0%	Cyprus
25.4%	31.1%	20.1%	15+	56.7%	47.0%	Czech Republic
28.0%	31.0%	25.0%	15+	50.7%	37.5%	Denmark
42.5%	75.0%	10.0%	13+	17.6%	28.8%	Djibouti
–	–	–	–	61.5%	74.4%	Dominica

Table A **Risk factors for cancer**

Countries	1 Population thousands	2 Youth smoking prevalence percentages (national data)	
		male	female
Dominican Republic	8,739	–	–
Ecuador	13,008	–	–
Egypt	67,559	6.3%	2.5%
El Salvador	6,533	12.7%	3.2%
Equatorial Guinea	494	–	–
Eritrea	4,390	–	–
Estonia	1,353	30.4%	18.2%
Ethiopia	68,613	–	–
Fiji	835	10.2%	5.3%
Finland	5,212	28.3%	32.2%
France	59,762	26.0%	26.7%
Gabon	1,344	–	–
Gambia	1,421	–	–
Georgia	5,126	32.7%	8.6%
Germany	82,541	32.2%	33.7%
Ghana	20,669	2.6%	1.4%
Greece	11,033	13.5%	14.1%
Grenada	105	1.8%	1.4%
Guatemala	12,307	–	–
Guinea	7,909	–	–
Guinea-Bissau	1,489	–	–
Guyana	769	2.0%	3.5%
Haiti	8,440	–	–
Honduras	6,969	17.1%	13.5%
Hong Kong SAR	6,816	–	–
Hungary	10,128	28.2%	25.8%
Iceland	289	–	–
India	1,064,399	6.6%	1.1%
Indonesia	214,674	–	–
Iran, Isl. Rep.	66,392	2.4%	0.0%
Iraq	24,700	–	–
Ireland	3,994	19.5%	20.5%
Israel	6,688	16.9%	11.6%
Italy	57,646	21.8%	24.9%
Jamaica	2,643	6.6%	4.2%
Japan	127,573	11.0%	5.0%
Jordan	5,308	16.6%	5.1%
Kazakhstan	14,878	14.2%	8.6%
Kenya	31,916	7.6%	3.8%
Kiribati	96	–	–
Korea, Dem. People's Rep. of	22,612	–	–
Korea, Republic of	47,912	–	–
Kuwait	2,396	13.1%	3.7%
Kyrgyzstan	5,052	9.1%	2.7%
Lao People's Dem. Rep.	5,660	–	–
Latvia	2,321	28.9%	21.1%
Lebanon	4,498	5.8%	2.2%
Lesotho	1,793	11.4%	5.0%

3 Adult smoking prevalence				4 Overweight prevalence		Countries
percentages			Age span	percentages		
total	male	female	years	male	female	
13.4%	15.8%	10.9%	18+	42.5%	62.8%	Dominican Republic
31.1%	45.5%	17.4%	18+	40.2%	50.9%	Ecuador
28.8%	45.4%	12.1%	20+	64.5%	69.7%	Egypt
25.0%	38.0%	12.0%	18+	42.1%	52.3%	El Salvador
–	–	–	–	35.4%	46.1%	Equatorial Guinea
7.2%	–	–	–	2.9%	5.9%	Eritrea
28.9%	45.0%	17.9%	16–64	50.7%	33.8%	Estonia
3.1%	5.9%	0.3%	18+	7.4%	3.1%	Ethiopia
15.0%	26.0%	3.9%	15–85	42.7%	63.4%	Fiji
22.2%	25.7%	19.3%	15+	63.8%	52.0%	Finland
25.4%	30.0%	21.2%	15+	44.1%	33.4%	France
–	–	–	–	22.7%	45.0%	Gabon
21.5%	38.5%	4.4%	15+	9.0%	20.5%	Gambia
27.8%	53.3%	6.3%	18+	37.4%	48.9%	Georgia
32.5%	37.3%	28.0%	18+	63.7%	53.6%	Germany
4.1%	7.4%	0.7%	18+	27.3%	26.2%	Ghana
37.6%	46.8%	29.0%	–	74.6%	60.1%	Greece
–	–	–	–	47.4%	56.4%	Grenada
11.0%	21.0%	2.0%	13–87	53.2%	61.1%	Guatemala
57.6%	58.9%	47.3%	11–72	14.5%	27.8%	Guinea
–	–	–	–	10.5%	20.3%	Guinea-Bissau
–	–	–	–	40.6%	51.2%	Guyana
10.4%	14.6%	6.1%	20+	13.0%	39.8%	Haiti
24.0%	36.0%	11.0%	18+	36.2%	47.5%	Honduras
12.8%	22.0%	3.5%	15+	–	–	Hong Kong SAR
33.8%	40.5%	27.8%	18+	55.9%	47.4%	Hungary
22.4%	25.4%	19.6%	15+	57.7%	60.5%	Iceland
31.7%	46.6%	16.8%	18+	15.0%	13.7%	India
28.7%	58.3%	2.9%	15+	9.6%	20.3%	Indonesia
10.6%	22.0%	2.1%	15+	47.3%	55.7%	Iran, Isl. Rep.
22.5%	40.0%	5.0%	16+	38.7%	49.0%	Iraq
27.0%	28.0%	26.0%	18+	50.0%	40.3%	Ireland
23.8%	31.9%	17.8%	15+	55.9%	56.3%	Israel
24.0%	31.3%	17.2%	15+	51.9%	37.8%	Italy
22.5%	37.7%	11.6%	25+	36.0%	71.8%	Jamaica
29.6%	46.9%	14.5%	20+	25.3%	18.6%	Japan
29.8%	50.5%	8.3%	18+	57.5%	67.3%	Jordan
37.3%	65.3%	9.3%	18+	43.9%	41.9%	Kazakhstan
11.2%	21.3%	1.0%	18+	6.5%	21.3%	Kenya
44.4%	56.5%	32.3%	16+	71.4%	71.9%	Kiribati
42.0%	–	–	–	31.0%	44.0%	Korea, Dem. People's Rep. of
34.7%	64.9%	4.4%	20+	32.8%	38.2%	Korea, Republic of
17.0%	34.4%	1.9%	18–60	69.5%	76.6%	Kuwait
25.4%	51.0%	4.5%	18+	34.5%	43.9%	Kyrgyzstan
–	58.7%	12.5%	18+	30.4%	43.5%	Lao People's Dem. Rep.
33.2%	51.1%	19.2%	15–64	49.9%	44.7%	Latvia
35.7%	42.3%	30.6%	25–65	51.7%	52.9%	Lebanon
19.8%	38.5%	1.0%	15+	26.3%	68.7%	Lesotho

Risk factors for cancer

Countries	1 Population thousands	2 Youth smoking prevalence percentages (national data)	
		male	female
Liberia	3,374	–	–
Libyan Arab Jamahiriya	5,559	2.0%	0.5%
Lithuania	3,454	34.9%	17.9%
Luxembourg	448	–	–
Macedonia, Former Yugos. Rep. Of	2,049	14.6%	12.7%
Madagascar	16,894	–	–
Malawi	10,962	–	–
Malaysia	24,774	–	–
Maldives	293	–	–
Mali	11,652	–	–
Malta	399	16.9%	17.4%
Marshall Islands	53	–	–
Mauritania	2,848	16.1%	4.7%
Mauritius	1,222	20.8%	6.8%
Mexico	102,291	–	–
Micronesia, Federated States of	125	–	–
Moldova, Republic of	4,238	19.4%	5.2%
Monaco	33	–	–
Mongolia	2,480	14.3%	5.1%
Morocco	30,113	3.1%	0.4%
Mozambique	18,791	–	–
Myanmar	49,363	24.8%	2.8%
Namibia	2,015	–	–
Nauru	10	–	–
Nepal	24,660	4.9%	1.3%
Netherlands	16,222	22.5%	24.3%
New Zealand	4,009	–	–
Nicaragua	5,480	18.6%	5.9%
Niger	11,762	12.6%	6.0%
Nigeria	136,461	–	–
Niue	2	–	–
Norway	4,562	20.1%	26.6%
Oman	2,599	3.7%	1.9%
Pakistan	148,439	0.7%	0.1%
Palau	20	–	–
Palestinian Authority	3,367	–	–
Panama	2,984	7.6%	10.1%
Papua New Guinea	5,502	–	–
Paraguay	5,643	–	–
Peru	27,148	–	–
Philippines	81,503	10.0%	2.9%
Poland	38,196	19.3%	12.6%
Portugal	10,444	17.6%	26.2%
Qatar	624	–	–
Romania	21,744	–	–
Russian Federation	143,425	27.4%	18.5%
Rwanda	8,395	–	–
Saint Kitts and Nevis	47	1.4%	0.7%

3 Adult smoking prevalence				4 Overweight prevalence		Countries
percentages			Age span	percentages		
total	male	female	years	male	female	
–	–	–	–	27.8%	39.2%	Liberia
4.0%	–	–	–	47.6%	56.0%	Libyan Arab Jamahiriya
28.3%	43.7%	12.8%	20–64	62.3%	43.9%	Lithuania
33.0%	39.0%	26.0%	15+	53.0%	52.6%	Luxembourg
36.0%	40.0%	32.0%	15+	37.1%	57.4%	Macedonia, Former Yugos. Rep. of
–	–	–	–	12.9%	18.1%	Madagascar
–	20.5%	4.8%	18+	14.3%	21.6%	Malawi
–	43.0%	1.6%	18+	22.5%	34.2%	Malaysia
–	37.4%	15.6%	–	29.7%	45.7%	Maldives
–	–	–	–	12.8%	26.1%	Mali
23.4%	29.9%	17.6%	15+	70.2%	65.1%	Malta
–	–	–	–	39.1%	50.0%	Marshall Islands
–	–	–	–	27.5%	52.2%	Mauritania
16.6%	32.1%	1.0%	18+	35.6%	49.5%	Mauritius
8.8%	12.9%	4.7%	18+	64.6%	65.6%	Mexico
–	42.0%	–	–	91.5%	89.5%	Micronesia, Federated States of
15.7%	33.6%	1.8%	15+	33.3%	45.4%	Moldova, Republic of
–	–	–	–	58.0%	64.3%	Monaco
30.0%	52.4%	7.5%	35+	46.0%	65.8%	Mongolia
14.3%	28.5%	0.1%	18+	31.1%	53.0%	Morocco
–	–	–	–	8.7%	24.3%	Mozambique
24.3%	36.4%	12.2%	18+	27.8%	41.1%	Myanmar
16.2%	22.8%	9.6%	18+	11.6%	31.5%	Namibia
54.4%	49.8%	59.0%	25+	96.3%	92.0%	Nauru
36.3%	48.5%	24.0%	18+	7.7%	8.0%	Nepal
32.0%	35.8%	28.4%	15+	46.7%	42.6%	Netherlands
–	23.7%	22.2%	15+	65.2%	64.0%	New Zealand
–	–	5.3%	–	48.9%	62.9%	Nicaragua
35.1%	40.6%	11.3%	15–35	12.1%	19.6%	Niger
8.9%	15.4%	0.5%	15+	19.6%	29.6%	Nigeria
26.1%	37.5%	14.5%	15+	76.9%	83.8%	Niue
26.0%	27.2%	24.8%	16–74	53.3%	42.0%	Norway
8.6%	15.5%	1.5%	15+	43.4%	46.0%	Oman
16.0%	28.5%	3.4%	15+	16.7%	23.2%	Pakistan
–	14.0%	4.0%	20+	72.7%	81.0%	Palau
22.0%	40.7%	3.2%	adult	–	–	Palestinian Authority
12.9%	19.7%	6.1%	15+	45.2%	54.7%	Panama
37.0%	46.0%	28.0%	15+	29.2%	26.1%	Papua New Guinea
15.1%	23.4%	6.8%	18+	40.9%	51.4%	Paraguay
33.8%	52.5%	17.8%	20–49	50.8%	62.7%	Peru
24.1%	40.5%	7.6%	18+	21.7%	25.4%	Philippines
32.0%	40.0%	25.0%	15+	50.7%	44.3%	Poland
20.5%	32.8%	9.5%	15+	55.5%	47.6%	Portugal
–	37.0%	0.5%	adults	56.9%	62.9%	Qatar
20.8%	32.3%	10.1%	15+	37.7%	40.6%	Romania
35.1%	60.4%	15.5%	18+	46.5%	51.7%	Russian Federation
–	7.0%	4.0%	40+	6.8%	19.2%	Rwanda
–	–	–	–	50.7%	58.9%	Saint Kitts and Nevis

Table A **Risk factors for cancer**

Countries	1 Population thousands	2 Youth smoking prevalence percentages (national data)	
		male	female
Saint Lucia	161	4.3%	0.4%
Saint Vincent and Grenadines	109	5.1%	2.6%
Samoa	178	–	–
San Marino	28	–	–
Sao Tome and Principe	157	–	–
Saudi Arabia	22,528	3.3%	–
Senegal	10,240	7.9%	1.5%
Serbia and Montenegro	8,104	–	–
Seychelles	84	16.0%	10.8%
Sierra Leone	5,337	–	–
Singapore	4,250	11.3%	7.7%
Slovakia	5,390	31.3%	27.1%
Slovenia	1,995	27.9%	30.2%
Solomon Islands	457	–	–
Somalia	9,626	–	–
South Africa	45,829	14.8%	8.3%
Spain	41,101	23.6%	32.3%
Sri Lanka	19,232	1.7%	0.7%
Sudan	33,546	9.8%	0.3%
Suriname	438	11.0%	3.3%
Swaziland	1,106	–	–
Sweden	8,956	11.1%	19.0%
Switzerland	7,350	25.4%	24.1%
Syrian Arab Republic	17,384	7.3%	2.7%
Tajikistan	6,305	–	–
Tanzania, United Republic of	35,889	5.9%	2.2%
Thailand	62,014	–	–
Timor-Leste	877	–	–
Togo	4,861	7.4%	1.4%
Tonga	102	–	–
Trinidad and Tobago	1,313	9.1%	1.6%
Tunisia	9,895	14.5%	1.1%
Turkey	70,712	11.2%	3.1%
Turkmenistan	4,864	–	–
Tuvalu	10	–	–
Uganda	25,280	–	–
Ukraine	48,356	44.6%	22.8%
United Arab Emirates	4,041	8.6%	1.0%
United Kingdom	59,329	–	–
United States of America	290,810	17.5%	12.3%
Uruguay	3,380	–	–
Uzbekistan	25,590	–	–
Vanuatu	210	–	–
Venezuela	25,674	5.4%	5.8%
Viet Nam	81,314	–	–
Yemen	19,173	4.0%	1.7%
Zambia	10,744	–	–
Zimbabwe	11,635	–	–

3 Adult smoking prevalence			Age span	4 Overweight prevalence		Countries
percentages				percentages		
total	male	female	years	male	female	
19.9%	37.3%	5.6%	25+	41.3%	65.7%	Saint Lucia
8.6%	17.4%	1.9%	19+	44.3%	54.0%	Saint Vincent and Grenadines
42.0%	60.0%	24.0%	29+	77.2%	80.7%	Samoa
22.7%	28.0%	17.0%	14+	57.6%	64.1%	San Marino
44.1%	–	–	–	14.4%	25.2%	Sao Tome and Principe
9.3%	14.4%	4.9%	30+	62.4%	63.0%	Saudi Arabia
32.0%	–	–	–	14.4%	34.1%	Senegal
40.4%	48.0%	33.6%	–	61.2%	48.5%	Serbia and Montenegro
–	37.0%	6.9%	12–64	55.1%	68.6%	Seychelles
21.5%	40.8%	7.4%	15+	20.2%	41.6%	Sierra Leone
13.7%	24.2%	3.5%	18–64	23.6%	20.7%	Singapore
32.0%	41.1%	14.7%	15+	50.7%	59.1%	Slovakia
23.7%	28.0%	20.1%	15–64	54.8%	62.1%	Slovenia
–	–	23.0%	15+	36.8%	48.0%	Solomon Islands
–	–	–	–	9.8%	19.3%	Somalia
15.5%	23.2%	7.7%	18+	38.2%	66.4%	South Africa
31.7%	39.2%	24.6%	16+	55.7%	45.7%	Spain
12.5%	23.2%	1.7%	18+	8.8%	5.0%	Sri Lanka
12.5%	23.5%	1.5%	adult	16.0%	27.0%	Sudan
–	–	–	–	41.0%	51.5%	Suriname
6.7%	10.5%	2.9%	18+	33.6%	45.2%	Swaziland
17.5%	16.7%	18.3%	16–84	51.7%	43.3%	Sweden
24.6%	26.5%	23.1%	15+	52.4%	53.8%	Switzerland
25.0%	44.3%	5.7%	25–41	47.2%	55.7%	Syrian Arab Republic
–	–	–	–	29.2%	41.8%	Tajikistan
25.5%	23.0%	1.3%	25–64	14.7%	32.5%	Tanzania, United Republic of
25.7%	48.5%	2.9%	15+	27.7%	46.4%	Thailand
–	–	1.1%	20+	35.9%	28.3%	Timor-Leste
–	–	–	–	15.0%	90.9%	Togo
31.7%	52.9%	10.5%	15+	89.5%	74.4%	Tonga
23.3%	42.4%	4.2%	35–74	54.8%	57.9%	Trinidad and Tobago
26.0%	49.5%	2.4%	18+	42.8%	65.4%	Tunisia
31.2%	49.4%	17.6%	15+	47.9%	45.5%	Turkey
14.0%	27.0%	1.0%	18+	48.1%	59.2%	Turkmenistan
41.0%	51.0%	31.0%	20+	51.2%	20.1%	Tuvalu
14.3%	25.2%	3.3%	–	6.9%	48.5%	Uganda
31.8%	52.5%	11.1%	18+	41.2%	68.4%	Ukraine
9.3%	17.3%	1.3%	18+	66.9%	58.8%	United Arab Emirates
26.0%	27.0%	25.0%	16+	62.5%	26.0%	United Kingdom
21.6%	24.1%	19.2%	18+	72.2%	69.8%	United States of America
29.2%	34.6%	23.8%	18+	60.0%	54.1%	Uruguay
12.5%	24.1%	0.9%	–	42.0%	44.3%	Uzbekistan
27.1%	49.1%	5.0%	20+	54.0%	60.1%	Vanuatu
28.7%	35.9%	21.4%	20–89	65.6%	57.5%	Venezuela
18.5%	35.3%	1.7%	18+	2.7%	7.0%	Viet Nam
53.0%	77.0%	29.0%	adult	24.6%	27.8%	Yemen
8.5%	16.0%	1.0%	–	7.0%	20.2%	Zambia
11.1%	20.0%	2.2%	18+	14.5%	47.2%	Zimbabwe

Statistics on cancer

Countries	1 The risk of getting cancer Probability of developing a cancer before age 65 percentages	2 Cancer survivors Five-year cancer survivors as a proportion of the nation's population survivors per 1,000 people	3 Primary prevention Percentage of infants given the 3-series hepatitis B vaccination (HBV)
Afghanistan	7.2%	1.5	–
Albania	13.0%	5.5	97.2%
Algeria	5.7%	1.1	–
Angola	7.8%	1.1	–
Antigua and Barbuda	–	–	99.0%
Argentina	12.5%	5.2	–
Armenia	12.0%	4.3	93.2%
Australia	15.2%	12.7	95.0%
Austria	13.9%	13.9	83.2%
Azerbaijan	9.7%	2.9	97.8%
Bahrain	6.7%	2.0	98.0%
Bangladesh	6.6%	1.4	56.0%
Barbados	10.1%	5.4	91.0%
Belarus	12.3%	6.5	90.5%
Belgium	15.1%	14.7	–
Belize	10.5%	2.7	95.8%
Benin	6.8%	0.9	81.0%
Bhutan	7.0%	1.6	95.0%
Bolivia	10.0%	2.8	95.1%
Bosnia and Herzegovina	13.6%	8.2	–
Botswana	9.7%	1.5	78.0%
Brazil	10.3%	3.4	91.0%
Brunei Darussalam	7.9%	2.1	–
Bulgaria	11.1%	6.7	95.8%
Burkina Faso	7.1%	0.9	–
Burundi	12.0%	1.5	–
Cambodia	7.8%	1.6	–
Cameroon	8.3%	1.2	–
Canada	14.7%	14.0	–
Cape Verde	6.6%	0.9	59.0%
Central African Rep.	8.7%	1.3	–
Chad	7.6%	1.0	–
Chile	10.4%	4.1	–
China	9.4%	2.4	96.7%
Colombia	10.2%	3.2	92.9%
Comoros	8.8%	1.3	27.0%
Congo	5.5%	1.0	–
Congo, Dem. Rep.	8.9%	0.8	–
Cook Islands	–	–	93.0%
Costa Rica	8.0%	2.6	86.2%
Côte d'Ivoire	6.9%	1.1	48.0%
Croatia	15.0%	11.2	97.9%
Cuba	7.6%	3.7	99.0%
Cyprus	10.4%	5.9	88.4%
Czech Republic	14.6%	10.7	67.0%
Denmark	14.0%	12.2	–
Djibouti	9.3%	1.6	–
Dominica	–	–	–

Incidence of cancer

per 100,000 people

male				female				Countries
lung	liver	oesophagus	testis	lung	breast	stomach	cervix	
12.2	3.7	10.3	0.9	2.9	26.8	9.7	6.9	Afghanistan
58.9	5.3	2.9	3.8	13.1	57.4	6.9	25.2	Albania
16.9	0.8	0.8	0.4	2.0	23.5	3.2	15.6	Algeria
7.1	5.3	6.2	0.4	1.3	23.1	9.7	28.6	Angola
–	–	–	–	–	–	–	–	Antigua and Barbuda
43.3	3.5	9.0	4.2	8.0	73.9	6.0	23.2	Argentina
58.9	4.2	2.7	3.1	7.5	51.6	9.9	16.8	Armenia
39.5	3.8	5.4	5.6	16.8	83.2	4.1	6.9	Australia
42.6	7.9	4.8	8.8	14.3	70.5	8.6	10.9	Austria
33.0	3.2	11.5	3.1	6.1	31.5	15.6	8.2	Azerbaijan
30.5	4.2	2.7	0.4	13.3	40.2	5.8	8.5	Bahrain
22.4	1.3	6.9	0.9	3.5	16.6	1.0	27.6	Bangladesh
15.3	2.9	10.6	0.8	3.2	62.4	6.7	24.9	Barbados
65.6	5.0	5.5	1.8	4.5	36.0	16.9	13.1	Belarus
75.3	4.2	6.8	5.0	12.2	92.0	4.8	9.3	Belgium
21.2	3.6	3.7	0.1	3.6	29.8	12.0	52.4	Belize
2.4	15.3	1.3	0.4	0.6	28.1	3.6	29.3	Benin
11.9	2.6	8.1	0.7	2.4	21.8	3.5	26.4	Bhutan
12.6	3.6	3.2	5.3	3.3	24.7	8.3	55.0	Bolivia
63.0	5.8	3.9	4.7	13.2	58.9	8.1	21.3	Bosnia and Herzegovina
8.7	4.5	9.0	1.3	3.0	33.3	2.2	30.4	Botswana
21.5	3.4	8.5	1.3	7.1	46.0	8.8	23.4	Brazil
24.3	9.5	3.1	0.9	11.6	20.6	6.4	18.7	Brunei Darussalam
45.6	4.9	2.7	3.2	6.7	46.2	9.2	18.7	Bulgaria
4.7	24.3	2.5	0.3	2.2	30.6	3.7	23.4	Burkina Faso
3.6	21.1	19.1	0.7	2.2	19.5	5.5	42.7	Burundi
22.5	15.0	4.6	1.0	4.9	21.5	5.1	38.7	Cambodia
3.0	41.3	0.7	0.5	0.4	29.7	2.9	35.7	Cameroon
55.8	4.0	4.4	4.6	31.6	84.3	4.0	7.7	Canada
2.4	15.3	1.3	0.4	0.6	28.1	3.6	29.3	Cape Verde
4.7	27.8	1.5	0.6	0.7	16.5	12.6	28.0	Central African Rep.
4.7	27.8	1.5	0.6	0.7	16.5	12.6	28.0	Chad
26.1	4.3	8.6	7.2	9.4	43.9	17.7	25.8	Chile
42.4	37.9	27.4	0.4	19.0	18.7	19.2	6.8	China
20.2	3.3	4.7	2.5	10.1	30.3	20.3	36.4	Colombia
3.6	21.1	19.1	0.7	2.2	19.5	5.5	42.7	Comoros
4.5	16.3	0.5	0.5	0.6	20.6	1.3	30.5	Congo
3.8	30.1	0.5	0.7	0.5	10.3	17.8	25.1	Congo, Dem. Rep.
–	–	–	–	–	–	–	–	Cook Islands
12.5	5.4	3.4	2.0	5.3	30.9	22.1	21.5	Costa Rica
6.1	12.8	1.2	0.6	1.2	26.0	3.6	30.1	Côte d'Ivoire
76.4	7.3	5.9	5.5	12.7	62.2	10.6	13.3	Croatia
40.0	4.3	4.8	0.6	16.3	31.2	4.3	20.2	Cuba
26.8	3.9	1.7	4.5	5.7	67.2	4.3	11.6	Cyprus
66.1	7.2	5.3	6.8	13.3	58.4	7.8	16.2	Czech Republic
45.3	4.3	5.8	10.3	29.7	88.7	3.8	12.6	Denmark
3.6	21.1	19.1	0.7	2.2	19.5	5.5	42.7	Djibouti
–	–	–	–	–	–	–	–	Dominica

Table B **Statistics on cancer**

Countries	1 **The risk of getting cancer** Probability of developing a cancer before age 65 percentages	2 **Cancer survivors** Five-year cancer survivors as a proportion of the nation's population survivors per 1,000 people	3 **Primary prevention** Percentage of infants given the 3-series hepatitis B vaccination (HBV)
Dominican Republic	9.2%	3.0	75.0%
Ecuador	7.9%	2.5	58.4%
Egypt	5.8%	1.0	97.7%
El Salvador	8.3%	2.4	88.1%
Equatorial Guinea	7.6%	1.1	–
Eritrea	8.9%	1.4	75.0%
Estonia	13.1%	8.3	95.9%
Ethiopia	10.0%	1.6	–
Fiji	6.8%	1.8	92.0%
Finland	11.9%	12.1	–
France	16.0%	13.8	29.0%
Gabon	8.1%	1.7	–
Gambia	5.6%	0.7	90.0%
Georgia	10.4%	4.7	48.6%
Germany	14.5%	14.4	81.0%
Ghana	6.8%	1.1	80.0%
Greece	10.3%	8.9	–
Grenada	–	–	97.9%
Guatemala	7.6%	1.8	–
Guinea	7.5%	1.0	–
Guinea-Bissau	6.7%	1.1	–
Guyana	9.0%	2.7	–
Haiti	8.9%	2.2	–
Honduras	7.6%	1.8	92.0%
Hong Kong SAR	–	–	–
Hungary	16.8%	10.6	–
Iceland	14.4%	11.8	–
India	6.6%	1.7	–
Indonesia	6.1%	1.8	75.0%
Iran, Isl. Rep.	6.2%	1.4	98.0%
Iraq	6.9%	1.5	–
Ireland	12.2%	9.1	–
Israel	15.3%	9.8	95.0%
Italy	13.8%	13.9	97.0%
Jamaica	9.5%	3.3	16.0%
Japan	10.1%	12.2	–
Jordan	7.2%	1.6	97.0%
Kazakhstan	14.6%	4.4	99.0%
Kenya	9.8%	1.4	73.0%
Kiribati	–	–	–
Korea, Dem. People's Rep. of	11.1%	3.3	99.0%
Korea, Republic of	11.1%	3.5	91.0%
Kuwait	5.2%	1.5	99.0%
Kyrgyzstan	9.8%	2.5	98.8%
Lao People's Dem. Rep.	6.4%	1.3	50.0%
Latvia	11.2%	7.9	98.1%
Lebanon	9.7%	3.1	88.0%
Lesotho	9.0%	1.5	17.0%

4 Incidence of cancer per 100,000 people								Countries
male				female				
lung	liver	oesophagus	testis	lung	breast	stomach	cervix	
18.6	7.9	3.4	0.9	9.3	36.1	9.2	30.8	Dominican Republic
10.5	5.9	2.9	3.8	6.1	23.5	27.0	38.7	Ecuador
8.6	6.1	1.5	0.2	2.8	24.2	2.0	9.7	Egypt
5.9	4.2	2.7	0.7	4.3	13.6	21.1	45.6	El Salvador
4.7	27.8	1.5	0.6	0.7	16.5	12.6	28.0	Equatorial Guinea
3.6	21.1	19.1	0.7	2.2	19.5	5.5	42.7	Eritrea
67.7	4.4	5.5	2.2	9.1	47.7	15.1	15.5	Estonia
2.7	19.3	28.1	1.2	3.2	24.7	5.1	35.9	Ethiopia
0.5	6.1	21.8	0.4	1.8	31.2	7.6	33.4	Fiji
33.4	3.4	3.5	3.2	10.1	84.7	6.0	4.3	Finland
52.6	10.5	11.0	6.7	8.8	91.9	4.1	9.8	France
9.9	11.7	3.6	0.3	1.7	18.2	0.6	30.6	Gabon
5.0	45.6	1.3	0.3	0.6	6.4	2.1	28.8	Gambia
37.2	7.6	2.6	2.2	7.2	51.8	9.1	17.5	Georgia
46.7	4.1	6.0	9.2	12.7	79.8	8.8	10.8	Germany
2.4	15.3	1.3	0.4	0.6	28.1	3.6	29.3	Ghana
58.0	12.9	1.6	3.0	8.7	51.6	5.9	7.7	Greece
–	–	–	–	–	–	–	–	Grenada
16.1	4.9	2.2	2.9	6.5	25.9	10.8	30.6	Guatemala
7.9	36.6	0.9	0.3	1.6	15.2	3.6	50.9	Guinea
2.4	15.3	1.3	0.4	0.6	28.1	3.6	29.3	Guinea-Bissau
7.5	1.3	2.5	2.2	5.0	29.5	8.8	47.3	Guyana
11.0	27.9	15.2	0.6	0.5	4.4	6.9	87.3	Haiti
16.1	4.9	2.2	2.9	6.5	25.9	10.8	30.6	Honduras
–	–	–	–	–	–	–	–	Hong Kong SAR
94.6	9.8	9.8	5.6	24.9	63.0	9.5	15.7	Hungary
30.0	2.1	5.3	5.9	30.0	90.0	6.6	8.3	Iceland
9.0	2.3	7.6	0.6	1.9	19.1	2.8	30.7	India
20.0	11.3	0.6	0.9	6.8	26.1	2.1	15.7	Indonesia
7.2	1.4	17.5	0.9	2.2	17.1	11.1	4.4	Iran, Isl. Rep.
22.7	0.9	1.2	0.8	6.7	31.7	3.8	3.3	Iraq
39.8	2.2	8.1	5.3	19.7	74.9	5.9	7.2	Ireland
27.2	3.3	2.3	3.8	11.3	90.8	6.9	4.5	Israel
58.0	15.9	4.1	2.9	10.7	74.4	9.7	8.1	Italy
24.1	4.1	5.1	0.7	6.0	43.5	11.6	31.2	Jamaica
38.1	23.1	10.0	1.5	12.3	32.7	26.1	8.0	Japan
16.5	2.5	1.4	1.4	3.5	33.0	4.0	4.2	Jordan
77.4	13.0	20.9	2.0	11.5	38.7	18.4	21.6	Kazakhstan
4.2	9.7	22.7	0.6	2.2	25.2	8.1	28.7	Kenya
–	–	–	–	–	–	–	–	Kiribati
53.3	47.1	8.9	0.5	12.8	20.4	26.8	17.9	Korea, Dem. People's Rep. of
53.3	47.1	8.9	0.5	12.8	20.4	26.8	17.9	Korea, Republic of
18.9	7.1	1.7	0.9	6.0	31.8	3.0	6.1	Kuwait
31.3	6.6	9.2	1.3	5.5	23.0	17.9	21.6	Kyrgyzstan
18.3	22.4	1.6	0.7	6.5	10.9	1.9	16.8	Lao People's Dem. Rep.
60.2	3.8	5.7	2.1	6.4	44.3	11.1	12.9	Latvia
31.3	0.8	1.4	1.5	5.0	52.5	4.6	15.4	Lebanon
11.6	23.7	16.4	0.7	1.6	13.1	2.2	61.6	Lesotho

103

Table B **Statistics on cancer**

Countries	1 The risk of getting cancer Probability of developing a cancer before age 65 percentages	2 Cancer survivors Five-year cancer survivors as a proportion of the nation's population survivors per 1,000 people	3 Primary prevention Percentage of infants given the 3-series hepatitis B vaccination (HBV)
Liberia	6.8%	1.0	–
Libyan Arab Jamahiriya	5.7%	1.0	–
Lithuania	11.6%	8.0	78.3%
Luxembourg	15.2%	13.5	49.0%
Macedonia, Former Yugos. Rep. Of	13.0%	7.5	–
Madagascar	9.0%	1.4	87.0%
Malawi	8.9%	1.1	–
Malaysia	8.1%	2.3	95.0%
Maldives	–	–	97.5%
Mali	7.4%	0.9	79.0%
Malta	11.7%	9.5	70.0%
Marshall Islands	–	–	74.0%
Mauritania	6.6%	1.0	–
Mauritius	6.6%	1.8	93.0%
Mexico	7.5%	2.3	97.9%
Micronesia, Federated States of	–	–	89.0%
Moldova, Republic of	12.6%	5.4	98.9%
Monaco	–	–	–
Mongolia	11.2%	1.5	97.8%
Morocco	5.7%	1.1	90.0%
Mozambique	8.8%	1.1	85.0%
Myanmar	8.4%	1.9	34.0%
Namibia	6.1%	1.1	–
Nauru	–	–	–
Nepal	7.0%	1.5	15.0%
Netherlands	13.9%	12.7	–
New Zealand	16.0%	13.1	–
Nicaragua	8.5%	2.0	86.0%
Niger	6.6%	0.8	–
Nigeria	6.7%	1.0	–
Niue	–	–	–
Norway	13.8%	13.4	–
Oman	5.6%	1.1	99.0%
Pakistan	9.1%	2.2	63.0%
Palau	–	–	–
Palestinian Authority	–	–	–
Panama	7.3%	2.7	86.0%
Papua New Guinea	9.8%	2.0	53.0%
Paraguay	8.4%	2.3	55.5%
Peru	10.3%	3.5	60.5%
Philippines	10.0%	2.5	–
Poland	14.1%	7.4	97.0%
Portugal	12.5%	10.0	94.2%
Qatar	8.0%	2.3	98.0%
Romania	11.4%	6.0	98.5%
Russian Federation	11.8%	5.8	93.6%
Rwanda	12.7%	1.5	96.0%
Saint Kitts and Nevis	–	–	99.0%

4 Incidence of cancer per 100,000 people								Countries
male				female				
lung	liver	oesophagus	testis	lung	breast	stomach	cervix	
1.6	9.8	1.6	1.2	0.6	18.7	2.0	35.0	Liberia
10.4	4.8	2.4	0.5	2.2	23.4	2.4	11.9	Libyan Arab Jamahiriya
57.5	3.2	6.9	1.4	5.6	38.5	13.0	17.5	Lithuania
61.3	4.2	7.7	7.6	13.6	82.5	6.7	8.7	Luxembourg
50.6	6.9	1.6	3.6	9.2	52.1	12.2	13.9	Macedonia, Former Yugos. Rep. of
3.6	21.1	19.1	0.7	2.2	19.5	5.5	42.7	Madagascar
2.5	4.8	16.4	0.2	0.4	10.5	0.8	46.6	Malawi
30.0	11.0	3.3	1.0	10.9	30.8	6.2	15.7	Malaysia
–	–	–	–	–	–	–	–	Maldives
2.8	29.7	2.9	0.6	0.1	18.2	19.5	35.2	Mali
41.1	3.3	3.8	3.1	6.1	76.1	5.0	4.8	Malta
–	–	–	–	–	–	–	–	Marshall Islands
2.4	15.3	1.3	0.4	0.6	28.1	3.6	29.3	Mauritania
15.7	3.0	4.2	0.3	5.1	31.6	6.7	18.2	Mauritius
17.0	5.0	2.2	3.1	6.7	26.4	9.4	29.5	Mexico
44.2	–	–	–	15.5	–	–	–	Micronesia, Federated States of
39.4	11.3	3.4	4.0	6.9	49.6	8.9	18.0	Moldova, Republic of
–	–	–	–	–	–	–	–	Monaco
31.8	98.9	24.5	0.2	11.3	6.6	23.3	18.0	Mongolia
20.1	1.3	0.8	0.4	2.0	22.5	3.1	13.2	Morocco
1.8	79.4	2.1	0.2	1.3	3.9	1.3	33.6	Mozambique
27.5	12.7	13.5	0.8	12.7	20.2	7.8	24.6	Myanmar
6.1	3.2	6.3	0.9	2.2	24.7	1.7	22.2	Namibia
–	–	–	–	–	–	–	–	Nauru
11.9	2.6	8.1	0.7	2.4	21.8	3.5	26.4	Nepal
59.7	1.8	6.9	5.8	17.8	86.7	5.2	7.3	Netherlands
37.3	4.6	5.9	6.4	20.5	91.9	4.5	10.0	New Zealand
12.2	6.0	2.1	1.3	5.4	23.9	17.6	47.2	Nicaragua
4.7	16.6	1.1	0.2	0.4	23.3	3.3	19.9	Niger
1.1	10.5	1.2	0.4	0.4	31.2	2.0	28.5	Nigeria
–	–	–	–	–	–	–	–	Niue
36.4	2.5	3.7	10.6	18.7	74.8	5.2	10.4	Norway
9.5	6.9	2.4	0.4	2.3	13.2	5.2	6.9	Oman
20.1	5.6	6.3	0.7	2.8	50.1	2.7	6.5	Pakistan
–	–	–	–	–	–	–	–	Palau
–	–	–	–	–	–	–	–	Palestinian Authority
15.0	2.8	2.0	1.9	5.6	29.0	9.6	28.2	Panama
2.2	19.4	2.9	0.6	1.3	17.3	2.9	40.4	Papua New Guinea
19.8	3.3	8.4	2.2	4.8	34.4	10.5	53.2	Paraguay
11.6	6.2	2.3	3.3	7.1	35.1	30.6	48.2	Peru
50.2	20.3	2.6	0.8	13.5	46.6	5.2	20.9	Philippines
82.0	3.6	6.0	4.1	14.6	50.3	7.8	18.4	Poland
34.2	5.6	6.5	4.6	6.0	55.5	13.6	13.5	Portugal
19.9	13.1	7.4	1.0	4.6	33.3	4.2	3.9	Qatar
50.0	10.0	2.9	3.2	8.5	44.3	6.8	23.9	Romania
66.8	4.6	7.0	1.9	6.6	38.8	15.8	11.9	Russian Federation
1.7	45.4	11.5	0.4	0.9	8.8	13.0	49.4	Rwanda
–	–	–	–	–	–	–	–	Saint Kitts and Nevis

Table B **Statistics on cancer**

Countries	1 The risk of getting cancer Probability of developing a cancer before age 65 percentages	2 Cancer survivors Five-year cancer survivors as a proportion of the nation's population survivors per 1,000 people	3 Primary prevention Percentage of infants given the 3-series hepatitis B vaccination (HBV)
Saint Lucia	–	–	14.0%
Saint Vincent and Grenadines	–	–	31.0%
Samoa	10.2%	2.1	–
San Marino	–	–	96.3%
Sao Tome and Principe	–	–	43.0%
Saudi Arabia	6.9%	1.6	94.8%
Senegal	6.7%	0.9	–
Serbia and Montenegro	13.0%	8.2	–
Seychelles	–	–	99.0%
Sierra Leone	6.7%	1.0	–
Singapore	10.4%	4.7	92.0%
Slovakia	13.8%	7.8	98.6%
Slovenia	13.2%	9.6	–
Solomon Islands	11.6%	2.2	78.0%
Somalia	8.9%	1.2	–
South Africa	11.5%	2.1	94.0%
Spain	12.7%	11.3	83.0%
Sri Lanka	6.6%	2.2	99.5%
Sudan	5.8%	1.1	–
Suriname	7.5%	2.3	–
Swaziland	8.6%	1.2	95.0%
Sweden	13.1%	15.1	1.0%
Switzerland	14.0%	15.1	–
Syrian Arab Republic	9.7%	2.2	–
Tajikistan	6.1%	1.3	62.0%
Tanzania, United Republic of	10.1%	1.5	95.0%
Thailand	8.3%	2.1	96.0%
Timor-Leste	–	–	–
Togo	6.9%	1.0	–
Tonga	–	–	93.1%
Trinidad and Tobago	9.3%	3.9	76.3%
Tunisia	5.7%	1.2	92.0%
Turkey	6.8%	1.8	68.0%
Turkmenistan	8.9%	1.9	97.0%
Tuvalu	–	–	95.0%
Uganda	9.4%	1.5	63.0%
Ukraine	12.3%	6.4	76.9%
United Arab Emirates	6.9%	2.1	92.0%
United Kingdom	12.9%	11.2	–
United States of America	17.7%	16.5	91.9%
Uruguay	15.0%	7.2	91.2%
Uzbekistan	7.3%	1.6	98.9%
Vanuatu	7.1%	1.2	56.0%
Venezuela	8.2%	2.6	75.0%
Viet Nam	7.5%	1.7	78.0%
Yemen	6.9%	1.3	42.0%
Zambia	10.5%	1.3	–
Zimbabwe	11.3%	1.5	80.0%

4 Incidence of cancer per 100,000 people								Countries
male				female				
lung	liver	oesophagus	testis	lung	breast	stomach	cervix	
–	–	–	–	–	–	–	–	Saint Lucia
–	–	–	–	–	–	–	–	Saint Vincent and Grenadines
17.4	12.3	2.1	2.6	1.0	34.2	11.6	28.0	Samoa
–	–	–	–	–	–	–	–	San Marino
–	–	–	–	–	–	–	–	Sao Tome and Principe
10.3	14.5	3.7	1.0	2.8	24.7	3.5	4.6	Saudi Arabia
1.4	30.8	0.3	0.2	0.1	18.4	3.1	26.2	Senegal
60.4	5.0	3.1	3.8	13.8	58.4	6.0	27.3	Serbia and Montenegro
–	–	–	–	–	–	–	–	Seychelles
2.4	15.3	1.3	0.4	0.6	28.1	3.6	29.3	Sierra Leone
46.4	18.4	6.0	1.1	18.3	48.7	11.1	13.2	Singapore
67.5	6.5	9.3	3.6	9.4	48.0	7.8	18.5	Slovakia
57.1	5.3	5.5	8.6	13.9	58.9	8.9	16.1	Slovenia
16.1	18.5	7.5	0.7	5.6	29.8	6.2	42.8	Solomon Islands
3.6	21.1	19.1	0.7	2.2	19.5	5.5	42.7	Somalia
25.0	6.1	20.7	0.9	7.5	35.0	3.9	37.5	South Africa
55.8	9.2	6.1	1.9	5.4	50.8	7.2	7.6	Spain
9.9	1.1	8.9	0.8	1.7	23.6	0.9	17.2	Sri Lanka
1.0	6.7	6.8	1.5	0.8	22.5	2.5	15.4	Sudan
13.6	0.9	3.4	1.8	7.6	30.0	4.7	27.0	Suriname
9.6	20.6	13.8	0.6	1.4	12.3	2.0	58.9	Swaziland
21.1	3.7	3.6	5.8	14.4	87.8	4.3	8.2	Sweden
44.6	6.2	6.1	10.1	13.8	81.7	4.6	8.3	Switzerland
32.9	0.9	1.4	2.1	3.7	44.8	5.5	2.0	Syrian Arab Republic
9.4	4.0	7.1	1.3	3.7	13.2	15.3	9.9	Tajikistan
2.0	8.8	19.9	0.6	0.5	21.1	4.6	68.6	Tanzania, United Republic of
25.5	38.6	3.2	0.5	10.4	16.6	2.9	19.8	Thailand
–	–	–	–	–	–	–	–	Timor-Leste
2.4	15.3	1.3	0.4	0.6	28.1	3.6	29.3	Togo
–	–	–	–	–	–	–	–	Tonga
14.3	1.5	2.5	1.2	4.6	51.1	9.2	27.1	Trinidad and Tobago
27.8	2.5	0.9	0.5	1.9	19.6	3.0	6.8	Tunisia
47.7	2.6	2.1	1.3	5.3	22.0	6.4	4.5	Turkey
22.0	5.5	20.7	1.8	4.8	17.9	13.5	13.5	Turkmenistan
–	–	–	–	–	–	–	–	Tuvalu
3.3	6.2	12.9	0.5	2.1	18.3	5.6	36.3	Uganda
58.0	4.2	5.9	1.8	7.4	39.9	12.6	14.1	Ukraine
13.7	5.5	7.1	1.1	5.2	24.1	8.7	9.9	United Arab Emirates
48.1	3.3	9.6	6.5	24.9	87.2	5.5	8.3	United Kingdom
61.9	5.5	5.9	5.5	36.1	101.1	3.3	7.7	United States of America
60.0	1.6	11.1	6.0	6.6	83.1	7.2	18.8	Uruguay
17.1	4.1	11.3	1.4	4.9	17.3	8.6	10.7	Uzbekistan
13.6	21.3	0.0	0.0	6.4	24.0	7.7	21.7	Vanuatu
18.6	3.5	2.5	1.6	10.5	34.3	12.2	36.0	Venezuela
29.6	23.7	3.7	0.7	7.2	16.2	9.9	20.2	Viet Nam
4.1	12.9	8.4	0.5	3.7	35.1	3.3	8.0	Yemen
6.5	18.9	6.4	0.1	0.9	13.0	6.9	53.7	Zambia
12.3	25.7	18.1	0.4	5.9	19.0	9.6	52.1	Zimbabwe

SOURCES

Please note that some figures in tables and graphs throughout the atlas may not appear to sum due to rounding.
In the sources below, op cit. is used to refer to identical citations in the same numbered edition.

GLOSSARY
http://www.cancer.gov/dictionary/

PART ONE INTRODUCTION

1 Mechanism of tumour development

Quote
Available from:
http://www.brainyquote.com.

Text
American Cancer Society. What is cancer? Available from:
http://www.cancer.org/docroot/CRI/content/CRI_2_4_1x_What_Is_Cancer.asp?area=.
National Cancer Institute. Dictionary of cancer terms under "cancer". Available from:
http://www.cancer.gov/dictionary.
Stewart BW and Kleihues P, editors. *World Cancer Report*. Lyon: IARC Press; 2003. p 84.
Murphy GP, Morris LB and Lange D, editors. *Informed Decisions*. New York: Viking Penguin; 1997. p 6-7.
National Cancer Institute. Dictionary of cancer terms under "tumor". op cit.
National Cancer Institute. Cancer facts, tumor grade: questions and answers. Available from:
http://cis.nci.nih.gov/fact/5_9.htm.
World Cancer Report. p 119. op cit.

How a tumour develops
Malignant transformation. In: Steinberg K, editor. *The Genetic Basis of Cancer* [book on CD-ROM]. New York: Oxford University Press; 2001.

How a tumour spreads
World Cancer Report. p 119. op cit.

Stage and prognosis
National Cancer Institute. Available from:

http://cis.nci.nih.gov/fact/5_32.htm. op cit.

Wow – not all cancers form solid tumours
American Cancer Society. What is cancer? op cit.
National Cancer Institute. Dictionary of cancer terms under "leukemia". op cit.

Wow – cancers that develop slowly Clipboard
World Cancer Report. p 84. op cit.

PART TWO RISK FACTORS

Part-title quote
http://www.worldofquotes.com/topic/Youth/2/index.html

2 Risk factors

Quote
Available from:
http://www.quotationspage.com/subjects/health.

Proportion of cancers caused by major risk factors
Dr D Maxwell Parkin, personal communication.
Stewart BW and Kleihues P, editors. *World Cancer Report*. op cit.
World Health Organization. Diet, nutrition and the prevention of chronic diseases. Geneva: WHO. *Technical Report* 2003; 916:95.

Wow – developing countries
World Cancer Report. p 56 (infections), p 33 (occupational carcinogens). opt. cit.

Growing obesity
WHO Global InfoBase team. *Surveillance of chronic disease risk factors: country-level data and comparable estimates*. Geneva: WHO. *SuRF Report* 2005;2.

Obesity and income
Sanmartin C, Ng E, Blackwell D, Gentleman J, Martinez M, Simile C. *Joint Canada/United States Survey of Health 2002-03*. Canada statistics catalogue no 82M0022XIE. Available from:
http://www.cdc.gov/nchs/data/nhis/jc

ush_analyticalreport.pdf. Accessed September 27, 2005.

Major modifiable risk factors
Tobacco use: Ezzati M, Henley SJ, Lopez AD, Thun MJ. Role of smoking in global and regional cancer epidemiology: current patterns and data needs. *Int J Cancer* 2005;116.
Unhealthy diet: *See text for* **7 Diet and nutrition**
Infectious agents: *See text for* **6 Infection**
Ultraviolet radiation: *World Cancer Report*. p53. op cit.
Physical inactivity: *Physical activity and health: a report of the Surgeon General*. Atlanta, GA: US Department of Health and Human Services, Centers for Disease Control and Prevention 1996.

Other modifiable risk factors
Alcohol use: *World Cancer Report*. p 29. op cit.
Occupational exposures: ibid. p 33-34. op cit.
Environmental pollution: ibid. p 39. op cit.
Obesity: Bergstrom A, Pisani P, Tenet V et al. Overweight as an avoidable cause of cancer in Europe. *Int J Cancer* 2001;91:421-30.
Food contaminants: *World Cancer Report*. p 43. op cit.
Ionizing radiation: ibid. p 51. op cit.

Non-modifiable risk factors
Ageing: USCS; Globocan; *World Cancer Report*. op cit.
Heredity: *World Cancer Report*. p 71. op cit.
Sex: *See* **10 The risk of getting cancer, Sex ratios of selected cancers**

Other risk factors
Reproductive factors: *World Cancer Report*. p 76. op cit.
Immunosuppression: ibid. p 68. op cit.
Medicinal drugs: ibid. p 48. op cit.

3 Risks for boys

Quote
Available from:
http://motivatingquotes.com/habit.htm and
http://www.stolaf.edu/people/robinso/russ261/dostoevsky/dostoevsky.html.

Text

Stewart BW and Kleihues P, editors. *World Cancer Report*. op cit.

Physical inactivity: *Physical activity and health: a report of the Surgeon General*. Atlanta, GA: US Department of Health and Human Services, Centers for Disease Control and Prevention 1996.

Preventing tobacco use among young people: a report of the Surgeon General. Atlanta, GA: US Department of Health and Human Services, Centers for Disease Control and Prevention 1994.

Global Youth Tobacco Survey Collaborating Group Differences in worldwide tobacco use by gender: findings from the Global Youth Tobacco Survey. *J Sch Health* 2003;73:207-15.

Rodgers A, Vaughan P, Prentice T, et al. *The World Health Report 2002*. Reducing risks, promoting healthy life. Geneva: WHO 2002;123-27.

Ross H. Economic determinants of smoking initiation and cessation. *Conference on public and private sector partnerships to reduce tobacco dependence*. Prague, Czech Republic: WHO Regional Office for Europe; 2001 Dec 13-14.

Diet, nutrition and the prevention of chronic diseases. WHO. op cit.

Currie C, Roberts C, Morgan A et al, editors. *Young people's health in context. Health behaviour in school-aged children (HBSC) study: international report from the 2001/2002 survey*. Geneva: WHO 2004;110.

Early starters

The GYTS is a collaborative project of WHO/CDC/participating countries (also include Associate Partners when data are used from countries in which they were involved). Analyses of GYTS data are not necessarily endorsed by WHO/CDC/participating countries.

J Sch Health. op cit.

Current GYTS data downloaded from http://www.cdc.gov/tobacco/global/GYTS.htm.

Currie C, Roberts C, Morgan A et al, editors. *HBSC*. p 67. op cit.

White V, Hayman J. Smoking behaviours of Australian secondary students in 2002. *National Drug Strategy Monograph Series No 54*. Canberra: Australian Government Department of Health and Ageing 2004.

Dr Yumiko Mochizuki-Kobayashi, personal communication, Aug 10, 2005.

Overweight boys

Cole TJ, Bellizzi MC, Flegal KM, Dietz WH. Establishing a standard definition for child overweight and obesity worldwide: international survey. *BMJ* 2000;320:1240.

HBSC. p 125. op cit.

Use of other tobacco products

J Sch Health. op cit.

Wow – overweight boys

HBSC. p 125. op cit.

4 Risks for girls

Quote

http://www.famous-quotations.com/asp/cquotes.asp?category=Children+%2F+Youth&curpage=2.

Text

J Sch Health. op cit.

Int J Cancer. op cit.

Calle EE, Rodriguez C, Walker-Thurmond K, Thun JM. Overweight, obesity, and mortality from cancer in a prospectively studied cohort of US adults. *N Engl J Med* 2003;348:1625-38.

Currie C, Roberts C, Morgan A, et al, editors. *HBSC*. p 90, 120, 128. op cit.

Stewart BW and Kleihues P, editors. *World Cancer Report*. p 84, 56, 144. op cit.

Vainio H, Bianchini F, editors. *IARC Handbooks of Cancer Prevention. Vol 5: Sunscreens*. Lyon: IARC Press; 2001.

Saraiya M, Glanz K, Briss P, et al. Preventing skin cancer: findings of the Task Force on Community Preventive Services on reducing exposure to ultraviolet light. *MMWR* 2003; 52:1-12.

Davis KJ, Cokkinides VE, Weinstock MA, O'Connell MC, Wingo PA. Summer sunburn and sun exposure among US youths ages 11 to 18: national prevalence and associated factors. *Pediatrics* 2002;110:27-35.

Early starters
Overweight girls
Use of other tobacco products
See **3 Risks for boys**

Wow – physical activity in children

HBSC. p 90. op cit.

5 Tobacco

Quote

http://edition.cnn.com/2005/WORLD/americas/02/07/cuba.smoking.ap/index.html. Accessed February 7, 2005.

Text

Ezzati M, Henley SJ, Lopez AD, Thun MJ. *Int J Cancer*. p 963-71. Table V – estimated cancer mortality attributable to smoking by site in the year 2000 and to other risk factors. op cit.

Ezzati M, Lopez AD. Regional, disease specific patterns of smoking-attributable mortality in 2000. *Tobacco Control* 2004;13:388-95.

The World Health Report 2002. Reducing risks, promoting healthy life. Geneva: WHO 2002;64.

International Agency for Research on Cancer. Involuntary smoking. IARC 2002;83. Available from: http://www-cie.iarc.fr/htdocs/monographs/vol83/02-involuntary.html. Accessed May 12, 2005.

Smoking prevalence among adults

SuRF Report. op cit.

WHO Regional Office for the Western Pacific. Available from: http://www.wpro.who.int/information_sources/databases/regional_statistics/rstat_tobacco_use.htm.

http://www.wpro.who.int/health_topics/tobacco.

http://www.wpro.who.int/media_centre/fact_sheets/fs_20020528.htm. Accessed August 4, 2005.

WHO Regional Office for Europe. Tobacco Free Initiative. Tobacco control database. Available from: http://data.euro.who.int/tobacco/. Accessed July 2005.

Smoking prevalence for men

The specific age ranges vary for different

countries, and are given in the tables.

WHO Global InfoBase team. *The SuRF Report 2. Surveillance of chronic disease risk factors: Country-level data and comparable estimates.* Geneva: WHO. 2005.

WHO WPRO. http://www.wpro.who.int/information_sources/databases/regional_statistics/rstat_tobacco_use.htm http://www.wpro.who.int/health_topics/tobacco http://www.wpro.who.int/media_centre/fact_sheets/fs_20020528.htm Accessed 04 August 2005.

WHO EURO. Tobacco Free Initiative. Tobacco Control database. http://data.euro.who.int/tobacco Accessed July 2005.

Afghanistan – Wielgosz AT. WHO assignment Afghanistan noncommunicable diseases CVD 1991.

Albania – *Evaluation of smoking prevalence among adult population.* November 2001. Institute of Public Health. Downloaded from WHO EURO Tobacco Control database.

Algeria – République Algérienne Démocratique et Populaire Ministère de la Santé et al. Mesure des facteurs de risque des maladies non transmissibles dans deux zones pilotes (approche STEPWISE) *Algérie 2003-Rapport.* 2004.

American Samoa – Mishra SI, Osann K, Luce PH. Prevalence and predictors of smoking behavior among Samoans in three geographical regions. *Ethnicity & Disease* 2005 Spring; 15(2):305–15.

Andorra – Health for All database. WHO EURO Tobacco Control database.

Argentina – Virolini M (Ministerio de Salud). *Encuesta Nacional de Tabaco 2004.* Ministerio de Salud y Ambiente de la Nacion.

Armenia – Gilmore A et al. Prevalence of Smoking in 8 countries of the Former Soviet Union: Results from the Living Conditions, Lifestyles and Health Study. *American Journal of Public Health* 2004. 94:2177–87.

Australia – Australian Institute of Health and Welfare 2005. *2004 National Drug Strategy Household Survey: First Results.* AIHW cat. no. PHE 57. Canberra: AIHW (Drug Statistics Series No. 13).

Accessed Sept 27, 2005. http://www.aihw.gov.au/publications/phe/ndshs04/ndshs04.pdf

Austria – Ulmer H et al. Recent trends and sociodemographic distribution of cardiovascular risk factors: results from two population surveys in the Austrian WHO CINDI demonstration area. *Wiener klinische Wochenschrift..* 2001. 113:573–9. Additional data from personal communication: Hanno Ulmer, Institute of Biostatistics, University of Innsbruck.

Azerbaijan – Adventist Development and Relief Agency et al. *Reproductive Health Survey.* Azerbaijan. 2001. Atlanta, US Department of Health and Human Services, 2003.

Bahamas – PAHO. *Tobacco or Health: Status in the Americas Pan American Health Organization.* 1992.

Bahrain – State of Bahrain. *The 2001 census of population, housing, buildings and establishments.* 2002.

Bangladesh – WHO World Health Survey.

Barbados – Cooper R et al. The prevalence of hypertension in seven populations of West African origin. *American Journal of Public Health.* 1997. 87:160–8. Additional data from personal communication: Richard Cooper.

Belarus – Health for All database. WHO EURO Tobacco Control database.

Belgium – Health for All database WHO EURO Tobacco Control database.

Benin – Fourn L and Monteiro B. Smoking and health in Benin. *World Health Forum* 1988;9:589–90.

Bolivia – Barceló A et al. Diabetes in Bolivia. *Pan American Journal of Public Health* 2001;10:318–23. Additional data from personal communication: Alberto Barceló.

Bosnia and Herzegovina – Noncommunicable disease risk factor survey: Federation of Bosnia and Herzegovina 2002; Ministry of Health of Bosnia and Herzegovina, Public Health Institute of Bosnia and Herzegovina. Downloaded from WHO EURO Tobacco Control database.

Botswana – WHO. *Tobacco or health: a global status report.* Geneva. 1997.

Brazil – WHO. World Health Survey.

Brunei Darussalam – Tobacco-Free Initiative Western Pacific Region. *Country Profiles on Tobacco or Health 2000.* WHO. WPR 2000. http://www.wpro.who.int

Bulgaria – *Health Interview Survey.* National Statistical Institute. WHO EURO Tobacco Control database.

Burkina Faso – Sondo B et al. Tabagisme des élèves des établissements secondaires du Burkina Faso. *Revue des Maladies Resporatoires* 1996;13:493-497.

Burundi – Mahwenya P. Analyse de la situation actuelle du tabagisme au Burundi. 1998.

Cambodia – National Institute of Statistics. *Cambodian Socioeconomic Survey* 1999. Phnom Penh: Author.

Cameroon – Cameroon smoking population. (2000). TMA – International Tobacco Guide (ITG). [CD-ROM]. Princeton, NJ: Author. http://www.tma.org/tma/products/Compendiums/itg.htm

Canada – *Canadian Tobacco Use Monitoring Survey Annual 2004.* http://www.hc-sc.gc.ca/hl-vs/pubs/tobac-tabac/ctums-esutc-2004/tabl01_e.html Accessed Sept 23, 2005.

Chad – Leonard L. Cigarette smoking and perceptions about smoking and health in Chad. *East African Medical Journal* 1996;73:509–12.

Chile – Ministerio de Salud de Chile. *Encuesta Nacional de Salud, Chile 2003.* Chile 2004.

China – China WHO WPRO database. Smoking Statistics. http://www.wpro.who.int/media_centre/fact_sheets/fs_20020528.htm Accessed August 28, 2005.

Colombia –Ministerio de Salud. *II Estudio Nacional de Factores de Riesgo de Enfermedades Cronicas.* Information provided by WHO PAHO Regional Office: April 29, 2003.

Congo – Kimbally-Kaky G et al. *Hypertension arterielle et les autres facteurs de risque cardiovasculaires à Brazzaville.* Brazzaville, Congo; 2004.

Cook Islands – Tobacco-Free Initiative Western Pacific Region. *Country Profiles on Tobacco or Health 2000.* WHO, WPRO, 2000. www.wpro.who.int

Costa Rica –Bejarano, J and Ugalde, F

(2003). *Estudio Nacional sobre consumo de drogas 2000-2001.* San José: I. A. F. A. Information provided by WHO PAHO Regional Office; April 29, 2003.

Cote d'ivoire –Schmidt, D, et al. En quete sur la consommation tabagique en milieu africain a Abidjan. *Poumon-Coeur* 1981;37: 87-94.

Croatia – *First Croatian Health Project, Sub-project on health promotion, the magnitude and context of problems – Baseline parameters.* Report, Zagreb. WHO EURO Tobacco Control database.

Cuba – Perez V et al. *National Survey of Risk Factors – 1995.* National Institute of Hygiene, Epidemiology and Microbiology, Ministry of Health and National Statistic Office; 1995.

Cyprus – *A household survey on smoking prevalence and behaviour in Cyprus.* Ministry of Health, Cyprus, 1997. WHO EURO Tobacco Control database.

Czech Republic – National Institute of Public Health. WHO EURO Tobacco Control database.

Denmark –WHO Health for All. WHO EURO Tobacco Control database.

Djibouti –Estimates made by Dr Abdillahi Hassan Hersi of the Ministry of Health in the unpublished report *Tobacco Related Problems in Djibouti,* submitted July 4, 1999.

Dominican Republic – WHO. World Health Survey.

Ecuador –Ockene, JK, Chiriboga, DE and Zevallos, JC. Smoking in Ecuador: prevalence, knowledge, and attitudes. *Tobacco Control* 1996;5:121–6.

Egypt – Herman WH et al. Diabetes mellitus in Egypt: risk factors and prevalence. *Diabetic Medicine,* 1995;12:1126–31. Additional data from personal communication: William Herman, MD, MPH.

El Salvador – PAHO. *Tobacco or Health: Status in the Americas* 1992.

Eritrea – Ministry of Health, Eritrea. National noncommunicable disease (NCD) risk factor baseline survey (using WHO STEPSwise approach).

Estonia – Health behaviour among the Estonian adult population (part of the international FinBalt Health Monitor survey – Finland, Estonia, Latvia,

Lithuania). WHO EURO Tobacco Control database.

Ethiopia – WHO. World Health Survey.

Fiji – Pryor J (FSM) et al. *Fiji NCD STEPS Report* (Draft) V4. 9.

Finland –Health for All database. WHO EURO Tobacco Control database.

France – Health for All database. WHO EURO Tobacco Control database.

Gambia – van der Sande MAB et al. Blood pressure patterns and cardiovascular risk factors in rural and urban Gambian communities. *Journal of Human Hypertension,* 2000;14:489–96. Additional data from personal communication: Marianne AB van der Sande.

Georgia – Prevalence of Smoking in 8 Countries of the Former Soviet Union: Results from the Living Conditions, Lifestyles and Health Study. *American Journal of Public Health* 2004;94(12):2177–87. WHO EURO Tobacco Control database.

Germany – Lampert, T and Burger, M Rauchgewohnheiten in Deutschland – Ergebnisse des telefonischen Bundes-Gesundheitssurveys 2003. *Gesundheitswesen.* 2004;66:511–17. WHO EURO Tobacco Control database.

Ghana – WHO. World Health Survey.

Greece – Kokkevi, A et al. , *Eur. Addict. Res.* 2000;6(1):42–49. Kokkevi, A et al. *Drug Alcohol Depend.* 2000;58(1–2): 181–188. WHO EURO Tobacco Control database.

Guam – Centers for Disease Control and Prevention, Prevalence of Current Cigarette Smoking Among Adults and Changes in Prevalence of Current and Some Day Smoking – United States, 1996–2000, *Morbidity and Mortality Weekly Report.* 2003;52;303–7.

Guatemala – Sakhuja R et al. Perceptions and prevalence of smoking among people in the highlands of Guatemala. *Cancer Causes and Control,* 2001;12:479–81.

Guinea –Ngom, A, Dieng, B and Bangoura, M. *Investigation of nicotine addiction in Guinea.* Conakry: Department of Health and Office of WHO in Guinea. 1998.

Haiti – Foundation Haïtienne de Diabète et de Maladies Cardio-Vasculaires.

Prévalence du diabète det de l'hypertension artérielle dans l'aire métropolitaine de Port au Prince, Haïti (PREDIAH 2003). Haiti, FHADIMAC; 2003.

Honduras – PAHO. *Tobacco or Health: Status in the Americas,* 1992.

Hong Kong – *General Household Survey, 2003.* Hong Kong Department of Health, Available online.

Hungary – WHO Health for All. WHO EURO Tobacco Control database.

Iceland – WHO Health for All. WHO EURO Tobacco Control database.

India – WHO World Health Survey.

Indonesia – Soemantri S et al. *National Household Health Survey Morbidity Study: NCD risk factors in Indonesia.* SURKESNAS 2001.

Iran, Islamic Republic of – Azizi F *Tehran Lipid and Glucose Study,* Endocrine Research Center, Shaheed Beheshti University of Medical Sciences, 2001.

Iraq – WHO. *Tobacco or health: a global status report.* Geneva: WHO; 1997.

Ireland – *The national health & lifestyle surveys 2002.* Health Promotion Unit, Department of Health and Children, 2003. WHO EURO Tobacco Control database.

Israel – WHO Health for All. WHO EURO Tobacco Control database.

Italy – WHO Health for All. WHO EURO Tobacco Control database.

Jamaica – Cooper R et al. The prevalence of hypertension in seven populations of West African origin. *American Journal of Public Health* 1997;87:160–8. Additional data from personal communication: Richard Cooper.

Japan – Higuchi S. *Survey on adult drinking patterns and prevention for related problems.* Ministry of Health, Labour and Welfare, 2004.

Jordan – Shehab F et al. Prevalence of selected risk factors for chronic disease – Jordan, 2002. *Morbidity and Mortality Weekly Report* 2003;52:1042–4.

Kazakhstan – Gilmore A et al. Prevalence of Smoking in 8 countries of the Former Soviet Union: Results from the Living Conditions, Lifestyles and Health Study. *American Journal of Public Health* 2004;94:2177–87.

Kenya – WHO World Health Survey.

Kiribati – Tobacco-Free Initiative Western Pacific Region. *Country Profiles on Tobacco or Health 2000*. WHO, WPRO, 2000. http://www.wpro.who.int

Korea, Democratic People's Republic of – WHO. *Tobacco or health: a global status report*. Geneva: WHO; 1997. Estimation of smoking in 2000; ERC Statistics International. *The World Cigarette Market*. Suffolk, UK, 2001.

Korea, Republic of – Suh IL. Cardiovascular mortality in Korea: a country experiencing epidemiologic transition. *Acta Cardiologica* 2001;56:75–81.

Kuwait – Memon A et al. Epidemiology of smoking among Kuwaiti adults: prevalence, characteristics, and attitudes. *Bulletin of the WHO*, 2000;78:1306–15.

Kyrgyzstan – Prevalence of Smoking in 8 Countries of the Former Soviet Union: Results from the Living Conditions, Lifestyles and Health Study. *American Journal of Public Health* 2004;94(12): 2177–87. WHO EURO Tobacco Control database.

Lao People's Democratic Republic – WHO World Health Survey.

Latvia – Health Behaviour among Latvian adult population, 2002. WHO EURO Tobacco Control database.

Lebanon – Soweid RA et al. *Together for heart health. An initiative for community-based cardiovascular disease risk factor prevention and control*. Nahhal Est 2002. Additional data from personal communication: Prof. Mustafa Khogali.

Lesotho – WHO *Tobacco or health: a global status report*. Geneva: WHO; 1997.

Libyan Arab Jamahiriya – General Secretary of Health and Social Welfare. *Tobacco Control in Libya*. 1997. Annual Report of the Center for Information and Documentation. Libyan Arab Jamahiriya.

Lithuania – Health behaviour among the Lithuanian adult population (part of the international FinBalt Health Monitor survey) WHO EURO Tobacco Control database.

Luxembourg –WHO Health for All. WHO EURO Tobacco Control database.

Macedonia, Former Yugoslav Republic of – WHO EURO Tobacco Control database.

Malawi – WHO World Health Survey.

Malaysia – WHO World Health Survey.

Maldives –*Smoking Survey 2001*. Department of Public Health Malé; 2001.

Malta –Health for All database, WHO EURO Tobacco Control database.

Mauritius – WHO World Health Survey.

Mexico – WHO World Health Survey.

Micronesia, Federated States of – Shmulewitz D. Epidemiology and factor analysis of obesity, type II diabetes, hypertension, and dyslipidemia (Syndrome X) on the Island of Kosrae, Federated States of Micronesia. *Human Heredity* 2001;51:8–19.

Moldova, Republic of – WHO EURO Tobacco Control database.

Mongolia – Suvd J et al. Glucose intolerance and associated factors in Mongolia: results of a national survey. *Diabetic Medicine* 2002;19:502–8.

Morocco – WHO World Health Survey.

Myanmar – WHO World Health Survey.

Namibia – WHO World Health Survey.

Nauru – Shaw J. Unpublished data for Nauru. 2003.

Nepal – WHO World Health Survey.

Netherlands –Health for All Database. WHO EURO Tobacco Control database.

Netherlands Antilles – *Curaçao Health Survey, 1993–94*, http://www.paho.org/english/sha/prfln er.htm Accessed 24 July 2005.

New Zealand – *A portrait of health – key results of the 2002/03 New Zealand Health Survey*. Wellington, Ministry of Health; 2004. Additional data from personal communication: Ministry of Health, New Zealand.

Nicaragua – Instituto Nacional de Estadísticas y Censos (INEC) et al. Encuesta Nicaragüense de demografía y salud 2001. Programa DHS+ and ORC Macro; 2002. Additional data from personal communication: Noureddine Abderrahim of ORC Macro.

Niger – Ministère Jeunesse Sports et Culture et al. Le tabagisme chez les jeunes au Niger. 1990.

Nigeria – **Males**: The National Expert Committee on NCD. Non-communicable diseases in Nigeria. Final report of a national survey. Federal Ministry of Health and Social Services; 1997.

Females: National Population Commission (NPC) [Nigeria] and ORC Marco. *Nigeria: Demographic and Health Survey 2003*. Calverton, Maryland, National Population Commission and ORC Macro; 2004.

Niue – Laugesen M. *Mission report on tobacco from Niue* 2003. Personal communication: Harley Stanton.

Norway – Interview survey, Statistics Norway; 2004. WHO EURO Tobacco Control database.

Oman – Sulaiman AJM et al. Oman family health survey 1995. *Journal of Tropical Pediatrics* 2001;47:1–33.

Pakistan – Pakistan Medical Research Council. *National Health Survey of Pakistan 1990–94* Network for the Rational use of Medication in Pakistan; 1998. Additional data from personal communication: AQ Khan of Pakistan Medical Research Council.

Palau –Palau Substance Abuse Needs Assessment (SANA) 1998.

Palestinian Authority – Smoking data from the Palestine Central Bureau of Statistics; Reported in *Country Profiles on Tobacco Control in the Eastern Mediterranean Region*. http://www.emro.who.int/TFI/Coun tryProfile. htm

Panama – Acción Latinoamericana Contra el Cáncer. 1998. Information provided by WHO PAHO Regional Office; April 29, 2003.

Papua New Guinea – Tobacco-Free Initiative Western Pacific Region. Country Profiles on Tobacco or Health 2000. WHO, Western Pacific Regional Office; 2000. http://www.wpro.who.int

Paraguay – WHO. World Health Survey.

Peru – *Encuesta Nacional Sobre Prevención y Uso de Drogas – Informe General, Perú 1999* – Instituto Nacional de Estadística e Informática – Contradrogas (Comisión de Lucha Contra el consumo de Drogas). Information provided by PAHO Regional Office April 20, 2003.

Philippines – WHO World Health Survey.

Poland – Nationwide survey on smoking behaviours and attitudes in Poland; 2000–2002. WHO EURO Tobacco Control database.

Portugal –WHO Health for All, WHO EURO Tobacco Control database.

Puerto Rico – "Do you smoke cigarettes now?"; Centers for Disease Control and Prevention. Behavioral Risk Factor Surveillance System. http://apps. nccd. cdc. gov/brfss.

Qatar – Smoking data from the Hamad Medical Center Survey; Reported in *Country Profiles on Tobacco Control in the Eastern Mediterranean Region.* http://www.emro.who.int/TFI/CountryProfile.htm

Romania – *Health Status of population in Romania*, Bucharest 2001, National Institute of Statistics. WHO EURO Tobacco Control database.

Russian Federation – Anna Gilmore et al. Prevalence of Smoking in 8 Countries of the Former Soviet Union: Results from the Living Conditions, Lifestyles and Health Study. *American Journal of Public Health* 2004;94(12): 2177–87. WHO EURO Tobacco Control database.

Rwanda – Currently smoking 5 or more cigarettes per day, two main hospitals of Butare; Newton R et al. Cancer in Rwanda. *International Journal of Cancer* 1996;66(1):75–81.

Saint Lucia – Cooper R et al. The prevalence of hypertension in seven populations of West African origin. *American Journal of Public Health* 1997;87:160–8. Additional data from personal communication: Richard Cooper.

Saint Vincent And Grenadines – Ministry of Health. Risk factor survey in St. Vincent. In: Pan American Health Organization/WHO; 1997.

Samoa – McGarvey ST. Cardiovascular disease (CVD) risk factors in Samoa and American Samoa; 1990-95. *Pacific Health Dialog* 2001;8:157–62. Additional data from personal communication: Stephen McGarvey.

San Marino – Current smoking in the early 1990s: *Tobacco or health: a global status report.* Geneva: WHO; 1997.

Sao Tome and Principe – Smoking at least one cigarette per day (survey year unknown); *Analise da Situacao do Tabagismo em S. Tome E Principe.* Organizacao Mundial da Saude, S. Tome; 1998.

Saudi Arabia – Saudi Heart Association. National cross-sectional study on coronary artery disease risk factors in Saudi Arabia (the CADIS study). 2001. Personal communication: Mansour Al-Nozha, Professor of Medicine and Consultant Cardiologist, Director, King Fahd Cardiac Centre.

Senegal – Kane A et al. Etude épidémiologique des maladies cardiovasculaires et des facteurs de risque en milieu rural au Sénégal. *Cardiologie Tropicale* 1998;25:103–7.

Serbia & Montenegro – Institute of Public Health of the Republic of Serbia "Dr Milan Jovanovic-Batut". *Health status, health needs and health care in Serbia*, Belgrade 2001 (WHO Survey). WHO EURO Tobacco Control database

Seychelles –Bovet P et al. The Seychelles Heart Study II: methods and basic findings. *Seychelles Medical and Dental Journal* 1997;5(1):8–24.

Sierra Leone – Lisk DR et al. Blood Pressure and hypertension in rural and urban Sierra Leoneans. *Ethnicity & Disease* 1999;9:254–63.

Singapore – *National Health Surveillance Survey 2001*. Ministry of Health; 2002.

Slovakia – WHO Health for All, WHO EURO Tobacco Control database.

Slovenia – Zakotnik-Mavcec J et al. WHO EURO Tobacco Control database.

Solomon Islands – Tobacco-Free Initiative Western Pacific Region. Country Profiles on Tobacco or Health 2000. WHO. WPRO; 2000. http://www.wpro.who.int

South Africa – WHO. World Health Survey.

Spain – National health survey 2001 (unpublished), Ministry of Health and Consumer Affairs. WHO EURO Tobacco Control database.

Sri Lanka – WHO World Health Survey.

Sudan – Smoking; Reported in *Country Profiles on Tobacco Control in the Eastern Mediterranean Region.* http://www.emro.who.int/TFI/CountryProfile.htm

Swaziland – WHO World Health Survey.

Sweden – WHO Health for All. WHO EURO Tobacco Control database.

Switzerland – Office fédéral de la statistique. Enquête suisse sur la santé. 2003. Additional data from personal communication: Marilina Galati-Petrecca, Division santè droit, èducation et science, Section de la santé.

Syrian Arab Republic – Maziak W et al. Smoking behaviour among schoolteachers in the north of the Syrian Arab Republic. *Eastern Mediterranean Health Journal* 2000;6:352–8.

Tanzania, United Republic of – Bovet P et al. Distribution of blood pressure, body mass index and smoking habits in the urban population of Dar es Salaam, Tanzania, and associations with socioeconomic status. *International Journal of Epidemiology* 2002;31:240–7.

Thailand – National Statistical Office et al. *The cigarette smoking and alcoholic drinking behavior survey 2001.* Bangkok, Thailand, National Statistical Office; 2002.

Timor-Leste – Estimated daily smoking; Barraclough S. Women and tobacco in Indonesia. *Tobacco Control* 1999;8: 327-332.

Tokelau – Reported in WHO WPRO Country Profiles, Tobacco or Health 2000. http://www.wpro.who.int

Tonga – Colagiuri S et al. The prevalence of diabetes in the Kingdom of Tonga. *Diabetes Care* 2002;25:1378–83.

Trinidad And Tobago – Miller GJ et al. Adult male all-cause, cardiovascular and cerebrovascular mortality in relation to ethnic group, systolic blood pressure and blood glucose concentration in Trinidad, West Indies. *International Journal of Epidemiology* 1988;17:62–9. Additional data from personal communication: George J Miller.

Tunisia – WHO World Health Survey.

Turkey – WHO Health for All, WHO EURO Tobacco Control database.

Turkmenistan – Piha T et al. Tobacco or health. *World Health Statistics Quarterly* 1993;46:188–94.

Tuvalu – Current smoking; Tuomilehto J et al. Smoking rates in the Pacific Islands. *Bulletin of the WHO* 1986;64(3): 447–56.

Uganda – Uganda Bureau of Statistics (UBOS) et al. Uganda Demographic and Health Survey 2000–2001. Calverton,

Maryland, UBOS and ORC Macro; 2001.

Ukraine – Gilmore A et al. Prevalence of Smoking in 8 countries of the Former Soviet Union: Results from the Living Conditions, Lifestyles and Health Study. *American Journal of Public Health*; 2004;94:2177–87.

United Arab Emirates – WHO World Health Survey.

United Kingdom – *Living in Britain: Results from the 2002 General Household Survey.* (Covering Great Britain only.) Office for National Statistics http://www.statistics.gov.uk/pdfdir/lib0304.pdf

United States Of America – Centers for Disease Control and Prevention. Cigarette smoking among adults – United States, 2003. *Morbidity and Mortality Weekly Reports* 2005;54(20):509-13

Uruguay – WHO World Health Survey.

Uzbekistan – Ministry of Health et al. *Uzbekistan Health Examination Survey 2002* – preliminary report. Calverton, Maryland, ORC Macro; 2003.

Vanuatu – Carlot-Tary M et al. *Vanuatu non-comunicable disease survey report.* Noumea, New Caledonia, Multipress; 1998.

Venezuela – Garcia-Araujo M et al. Factores nutricionales y metabólicos como riesgo de enfermedades cardiovasculares en una población adulta de la ciudad de Maracaibo Estado Zulia, Venezuela. *Investigacion Clinica* 2001;42:23–42.

Viet Nam – WHO. World Health Survey.

Virgin Islands (USA) – Centers for Disease Control and Prevention, State-Specific Prevalence of Current Cigarette Smoking Among Adults – United States; 2003. *Morbidity and Mortality Weekly Report* 2004;5;1.

Yemen – Sanaa University Survey by A Hadarani. Reported in *Country Profiles on Tobacco Control in the Eastern Mediterranean Region.* http://www.emro.who.int/TFI/CountryProfile.htm

Zambia – Pampel FC. Patterns of tobacco use in the early epidemic stages: Malawi and Zambia; 2000–02. *Am J Public Health* 2005;95(6):1009–15.

Zimbabwe – WHO World Health Survey.

Cancer deaths caused by smoking
Wow – cancer deaths
Clipboard
Int J Cancer. op cit.

Cancer and tobacco
Int J Cancer. op cit.
Ferlay J, Bray F, Pisani P, Parkin DM. Globocan 2002. Cancer incidence, mortality and prevalence worldwide. *IARC CancerBase No 5, version 2.0.* Lyon: IARC Press, 2004.

6 Infection

Text
Parkin DM. The global health burden of infection associated cancers in the year 2002. *Int J Cancer* (in press).

Helicobacter pylori
Brown LM, *Helicobacter pylori*: epidemiology and routes of transmission. *Epidemiol. Reviews* 2000; 22:283-97.
Eurogast Study Group An international association between *Helicobacter pylori* infection and gastric cancer. *Lancet* 1993.
Everhart J.E. Recent developments in the epidemiology of *Helicobacter pylori*. *Gastroenterol. Clinics of N America* 2002;29:559-78.
Go MF. Natural history and epidemiology of *Helicobacter pylori* infection. *Alim Pharm Ther* 2002;16: 3-15.
Helicobacter and Cancer Collaborative Group Gastric cancer and *Helicobacter pylori*: a combined analysis of 12 case-control studies nested within prospective cohorts. *Gut* 2001; 49:347-53.
IARC Monographs on the Evaluation of Carcinogenic Risks to Humans. Vol 61 schistosomes, liver flukes and *Helicobacter pylori*. Lyon: IARC Press, 1994.
Mégraud F, Brassens-Rabbé MP, Denis F, Belbouri A, Hoa DQ. Seroepidemiology of Campylobacter pylori infection in various populations. *Journal of Clinical Microbiology* 1989;27:1870-73.
Wang KJ, Wang RT. Meta-analysis on the epidemiology of *Helicobacter pylori* infection in China. *Zhonghua Liu Xing Bing Xue Za Zhi* 2003;24:443-6.

World cancer burden caused by infections
Infection as a cause of cancer
Parkin DM. *Int J Cancer.* op cit.
Regions as defined by World Population Prospects, Department of Economic and Social Affairs, United Nations. Available from:
http://esa.un.org/unpp/index.asp?panel=5.

7 Diet and nutrition

Quote
Available from:
http://www.topendsports.com/nutrition/quotes.htm.

Text
Doll R, Peto R. Epidemiology of cancer. In: Weatherall DJ, Ledingham JGG, Warrell DA, editors. *Oxford Textbook of Medicine.* Oxford: Oxford University Press;1996. p 197-221.
Willet MC. Diet, nutrition, and avoidable cancer. *Environmental Health Perspectives* 1995;103(supp 8):S165-70.
Vainio H, Bianchini F, editors. *IARC Handbooks of Cancer Prevention. Vol 5: sunscreens.* Lyon: IARC Press; 2001.
IARC Handbooks of Cancer Prevention. Vol 6: weight control and physical activity. Lyon: IARC Press; 2002.
World Health Organization. *Global Status Report on Alcohol.* WHO 2004.

Overweight
SuRF Report. op cit.

Strength of evidence on physical activity and dietary factors
Diet, nutrition and the prevention of chronic diseases. Report of a joint WHO/FAO expert consultation, January 28 – February 1, 2002. Geneva: WHO. *Technical Report* 2003; 916.

Meat consumption
Bruinsma J, editor. *World agriculture: towards 2015/2030. An FAO perspective.* Rome: Food and Agriculture Organization of the United Nations/London: Earthscan; 2003.

Dietary recommendations for reducing the risk of cancer
Diet, nutrition and the prevention of chronic diseases. Report of a joint WHO/FAO expert consultation. op cit.

8 Ultraviolet radiation

Text
IARC Monographs on the Evaluation of Carcinogenic Risks to Humans. Vol 55. Solar and Ultraviolet Radiation. Lyon: IARC Press, 1992.
http://www.acpm.org/skinprot.htm.
IARC Handbooks of Cancer Prevention. Vol 5. op cit.

Mean annual UV radiation level
World Health Organization/World Meteorological Organization /United Nations Environment Programme/International Commission on Non-Ionizing Radiation Protection. *Global Solar Index: A Practical Guide.* Geneva: WHO; 2002.
Unpublished data from Schmalwieser AW, Institute of Medical Physics and Biostatistics, University of Veterinary Medicine, Vienna, Austria by model calculations described in: Schmalwieser AW, et al. Global validation of a forecast model for irradiance of the solar, erythemally effective UV radiation. *Journal of Optical Engineering* 2002;40:3040-50.

Malignant melanoma of skin
Around 1995. Parkin DM, Whelan SL, Ferlay J, Teppo L and Thomas DB, editors. *Cancer Incidence in Five Continents, Vol VIII IARC Scientific publication 155*, Lyon: IARC Press; 2002.

Trends in malignant melanoma of skin
Parkin DM, Whelan S, Ferlay J and Storm H. *Cancer Incidence in Five Continents, Vol I to VIII. IARC CancerBase No 7*, Lyon, 2005.

9 Reproductive and hormonal factors

Text
Collaborative Group on Hormonal Factors in Breast Cancer. Breast cancer and hormonal contraceptives: collaborative re-analysis of individual data on 53,297 women with breast cancer and 100,239 women without breast cancer from 54 epidemiological studies. *Lancet* 1996;347:1713-27.
Collaborative Group on Hormonal Factors in Breast Cancer. Breast cancer and hormone replacement therapy: collaborative reanalysis of data from 51 epidemiological studies of 52,705 women with breast cancer and 108,411 women without breast cancer. *Lancet* 1997 Oct 11;350(9084):1047-59.
Million Women Study Collaborators. Breast cancer and hormone replacement therapy in the Million Women Study. *Lancet* 2003;362:419-27.
Rose PG. Endometrial Carcinoma. *N Engl J Med* 1996;335:640-49.
Whittemore AS, Harris R, Itnyre J, and the Collaborative Ovarian Cancer Group Characteristics relating to ovarian cancer risk: collaborative analysis of 12 US case-control studies. II. Invasive epithelial ovarian cancers in white women. *Am J Epidemiol* 1992;136:1184-203.
Muñoz N, Franceschi S, Bosetti C, et al. Role of parity and Human papillomavirus in cervical cancer: the IARC multicentric case-control study. *Lancet* 359(9312):1093-101.
Lane-Claypon JE. A further report on cancer of the breasts, with special reference to its associated antecedent conditions. *Report on Public Health and Medical Subjects No 32*. London: HMSO; 1926.
Collaborative Group on Hormonal Factors in Breast Cancer. Breast cancer and breastfeeding: collaborative reanalysis of individual data from 47 epidemiological studies in 30 countries, including 50,302 women with breast cancer and 96,973 women without the disease. *Lancet* 2002;360(9328):187-95.

Total fertility rates
World fertility patterns. New York: Population Division of the Department of Economic and Social Affairs of the United Nations Secretariat; 2004. Available from:
http://www.un.org/esa/population/pu blications/Fertilitypatterns_chart/Fertilit y_Patterns_wallchart.htm.

Oral contraceptives
IARC Monographs on the Evaluation of Carcinogenic Risks to Humans. Vol 72 hormonal contraception and post-menopausal hormonal therapy. Lyon: IARC Press; 1999.

Wow – contraceptive use
Available from:
http://www.cancer.gov/cancertopics/p dq/prevention accessed Sept. 30, 2005.

Risk of breast cancer
Lancet 1996;347. op cit.
Lancet 1997;350. op cit.
Lancet 2002;360. op cit.
Beral V, Bull D, Doll R, Peto R, Reeves G; Collaborative Group on Hormonal Factors in Breast Cancer. Breast cancer and abortion: collaborative reanalysis of data from 53 epidemiological studies, including 83,000 women with breast cancer from 16 countries. *Lancet* 2004 Mar 27;363(9414):1007-16.
Lancet 2003;362. op cit.

PART THREE THE BURDEN

Part-title quote
http://www.worldofquotes.com/search. php

10 The risk of getting cancer

Text
http://seer.cancer.gov/publicdata.
Parkin DM, Whelan SL, Ferlay J, Teppo L and Thomas DB, editors. *IARC Scientific Publication 155* op cit.

Cancer risk
Ferlay J, Bray F, Pisani P, Parkin DM. *IARC CancerBase No 5, version 2.0.* op cit.

Age-specific incidence
IARC Scientific Publication 155. op cit.

Sex ratios of selected cancers
IARC Scientific Publication 155. op cit.
http://www.cancerindex.org/clinks3m. htm. Accessed Dec 3, 2005.

11 Major cancers

Text

Parkin DM, Bray F, Ferlay J, Pisani P
Global cancer statistics 2002. *CA Cancer J
Clin.* 2005 Mar-Apr;55(2):74-108.

Sex differences
Differences around the world

Ferlay J, Bray F, Pisani P, Parkin DM. *IARC
CancerBase No 5, version 2.0.* op cit.

12 Geographical diversity

Quote

http://home.att.net/~quotesabout/hippo
crates.html. Accessed May 16, 2005

All maps

Ferlay J, Bray F, Pisani P, Parkin DM. *IARC
CancerBase No 5, version 2.0.* op cit.

13 Lung cancer

Quote

Available from:
http://www.worldofquotes.com.

Text

Ferlay J, Bray F, Pisani P, Parkin DM. *IARC
CancerBase No 5, version 2.0.* op cit.
Nafstad1 P, Håheim LL, Oftedal1 B, Gram
F, Holme I, Hjermann I, Leren P Lung
cancer and air pollution: a 27-year follow
up of 16,209 Norwegian men. Thorax
2003; 58:1071-76.
Harris JE, Thun MJ, Mondul AM, Calle
EE. Cigarette tar yields in relation to
mortality from lung cancer in the cancer
prevention study II prospective cohort
1982-8. *BMJ* 2004 Jan 10;328:72,
doi:10.1136/bmj.37936.585382.44.

Wow

*IARC Monographs on the Evaluation of
Carcinogenic Risks to Humans. Vol 83 tobacco
Smoke and inVoluntary smoking.* Summary
of data reported and evaluation. Available
from:
http://monographs.iarc.fr/htdocs/index
es/Vol83index.html. Accessed
September 26, 2005.

Lung cancer incidence

IARC CancerBase. op cit.

Trends in mortality from lung cancer

World Health Organization. WHO
Statistical Information System
(WHOSIS). Mortality database available
from:
http://www3.who.int/whosis/menu.cfm.

Trends in survival from lung cancer

Scotland: Scottish Health Statistics.
Available from:
http://www.isdscotland.org.
USA: Trends in lung cancer morbidity and
mortality. American Lung Association
Epidemiology and Statistic Unit.
Research And Program Services. May
2005. Available from:
http://www.lungusa.org.

14 Cancer in children

Text

Parkin DM, Kramárová E, Draper, GJ,
Masuyer E, Michaelis J, Neglia J, Qureshi
S and Stiller CA, editors. International
Incidence of Childhood Cancer Vol II.
IARC Scientific Publication 144. Lyon:
IARC Press; 1998.
Cancer Facts and Figures. Atlanta, GA:
American Cancer Society; 2005.
Ries LAG, Smith MA, Gurney JG, Linet
M, Tamra T, Young JL, Bunin GR,
editors. *Cancer Incidence and Survival
among Children and Adolescents: United
States SEER Program 1975-95.* Bethesda,
MD: National Cancer Institute, SEER
Program1999:NIH 99-4649.

Cancers in children

IARC Scientific Publication 144. op cit.

**Trends in the incidence of the major
cancers of children**
**Trends in the five-year survival of
children suffering from the major
cancers**

Steliarova-Foucher E, Stiller C, Kaatsch P,
Berrino F, Coebergh JW, Lacour B and
Parkin DM. Geographical patterns and
time trends of cancer incidence and
survival among children and adolescents
in Europe since the 1970s (the ACCIS
project): an epidemiological study.
Lancet 2004 Dec
11;364(9451):2097–105.

Clipboard

Stiller CA. Epidemiology and genetics of
childhood cancer. *Oncogene*
2004;23:6429-44.

15 Cancer survivors

Quote

Available from:
http://www.10ktruth.com/the_quotes/
cycle.htm. Accessed September 16, 2005.

Text

CDC, Lance Armstrong Foundation. A
national action plan for cancer
survivorship: advancing public health
strategies. Atlanta, GA: US Department
of Health and Human Services, CDC;
2004. Available from:
http://www.cdc.gov/cancer/survivorshi
p/overview.htm. Accessed September 9,
2005.
Parkin DM, Bray F, Ferlay J, Pisani P *CA
Cancer J Clin*; 55:74–108. op cit.
Living Beyond Cancer: finding a new
balance. *President's Cancer Panel 2003–04
Annual Report*; May 2004. Available at:
http://deainfo.nci.nih.gov/advisory/pcp
/pcp03-04rpt/Survivorship.pdf.
Accessed Sept 9, 2005.

Five-year cancer survivors

Available from: http://www-depiarc.fr,
accessed August 22, 2005
CA Cancer J Clin. op cit.

Symbol on map – Relay for Life

Darnelle Bernier, ACS, Manager of
International Relay For Life, personal
communication.
darnelle.bernier@cancer.org.

Wow – Europe

CA Cancer J Clin. op cit.

Wow – 24.6 million cancer survivors

Living beyond cancer: a European dialogue.
*President's Cancer Panel 2003–04 Annual
Report* (supplement); May 2004. Available
from:
http://deainfo.nci.nih.gov/advisory/pcp
/pcp03-04rpt/Supplement.pdf. Accessed
September 9, 2005.

Relay for Life
Available from:
http://www.cancer.org/docroot/GI/content/GI_1_3_Relay_For_Life_International.asp. Accessed August 28, 2005.

Number of cancer survivors
Available from:
http://dccps.nci.nih.gov/ocs/prevalence/prevalence.html#time. Accessed August 30, 2005.

PART FOUR ECONOMICS

Part-title quote
http://www.motivatingquotes.com/healthq.htm

16 Economic costs

Quote
Available from:
http://www.worldofquotes.com/author/Gerald-P-O'driscoll/1. Accessed June 15, 2005.

Text
Wagner L, Lacey MD. The hidden costs of cancer care: an overview with implications of referral resources for oncology nurses. *Clinical Journal of Oncology Nursing* 2004;8:279-86.
Organization for Economic Cooperation and Development (OECD). *A disease-based comparison of health systems: What is best and at what cost?* Paris: OECD; 2003.

USA and Canada
Herper M. *Cancer's Cost Crisis* June 2004. Available from:
http://www.forbes.com/technology/2004/06/08/cx_mh_0608costs.html. Accessed April 1, 2005.
Economic burden of cancer in Canada 1998. Available from:
http://www.cancer.ca/ccs/internet/standard/0,3182,3172_367655_379099048_langId-en,00.html.

Switzerland
Zurn P, Danthine J-P: Economic evaluation of different vaccination strategies against hepatitis B in Switzerland. *Soz-Präventivmed* 1998;1(suppl):S61–S64.

China
Liu ZG, Zhao SL, Zhang YX: Cost-benefit analysis on immunization of newborns with hepatitis B vaccine in Jinan City. *Chin J Epidemiol* 1995;16:81-4.

Sweden
Apoteket AB. Total drug sales in Sweden 2000-04, retail prices, VAT excluded – Statistics from the National Corporation of Swedish Pharmacies. Stockholm, Sweden; 2005. Available from:
http://www.apoteket.se/content/1/c4/48/05/auptot.pdf. Accessed May 18, 2005.

UK
Bosanquet N, Sikora K. The economics of cancer care in the UK. *Lancet Oncol* 2004;5:568-74.

France
Levy C, Bonastre J: The cost of chemotherapy. *Bull Cancer* 2003;90:976-82.

Chile
Tobacco and poverty: a vicious cycle. *Newsletter of the Pan American Health Organization*; Available from:
http://www.paho.org/English/DD/PIN/ptoday15_jul04.htm. Accessed March 19, 2005.

The Netherlands
Polder JJ, Achterberg PW. *Cost of illness in the Netherlands*. Bilthoven: National Institute for Public Health and the Environment; 2004.
A disease-based comparison of health systems: What is best and at what cost? op cit.

The cost of treating obesity
Finkelstein EA, Fiebelkorn IC, Wang G. State-level estimates of annual medical expenditures attributable to obesity. *Obesity Research* 2004;12:18-24.

The cost of breast cancer treatment
A disease-based comparison of health systems: What is best and at what cost? op cit.

Cost savings
Margolis H, Coleman P, Brown R, et al. Prevention of hepatitis B virus transmission by immunization. *J Am Med Assoc* 1995;274:1201-08.

Trends in cancer-related direct costs
Brown ML, Lipscomb J, Snyder C. The burden of illness of cancer: economic cost and quality of life. *Annu Rev Public Health* 2001;22:91-113.
National Heart, Lung, and Blood Institute (NHLBI). *NHBLI Fact Book Fiscal Year 2004*. Available from:
http://www.nhlbi.nih.gov/about/04fackbk.pdf. Accessed May 2, 2005.

The price of 100 packs of cigarettes
Wow – cigarettes are most affordable
Blecher EH, van Walbeek CP An international analysis of cigarette affordability. *Tobacco Control* 2004;13:339-46.

17 Commercial interests

Quote
Moses H III, Dorsey ER, Matheson DHM, Their SO. Financial Anatomy of Biomedical Research. *JAMA* 2005;294:1333-42.

Text
Mackay J. Commentary: lessons from private statements of the tobacco industry. *Bulletin of the World Health Organization* 2000;78(7):911–12.
Stewart BW and Kleihues P, editors. *World Cancer Report*. p 33-34. op cit.

Biomedical research
JAMA. op cit.

Profits from tobacco
Hoovers™ Available from:
http://www.hoovers.com. Accessed July 19, 2005.
JTI data for fiscal year ending March 2005. Japan Tobacco Inc Annual Report 2005, p7, 62. Available from:
http://www.jti.co.jp/JTI_E/IR/05/annual2005/annual2005_E_all.pdf, accessed July 19 and 22, 2005.
Philip Morris, Net Revenues, US Securities and Exchange Commission. Available from:
http://www.sec.gov/Archives/edgar/data/764180/000095012305003146/y06457exv13.htm. Accessed July 22, 2005.
BAT Annual Report 2004, Available from: http:www.bat.com. Accessed July 22, 2005.

Imperial, Annual Report 2004 Available from: http://www.imperial-tobacco.com/?pageid=185&subsection=restofweurope. Accessed July 22, 2005.

Gallaher Group, Annual Report 2004 Available from: http://ir.gallaher-group.com/ir/publications/index.asp?tag=on. Accessed July 22, 2005.

Altadis, Annual Report 2004, p iii, Available from: http://www.altadis.com/en/shareholders/pdf/meeting2005/infoanual2004.pdf. Accessed July 22, 2005.

Wow – 1 in 5 cancer deaths
Ezzati M, Henley SJ, Lopez AD, Thun MJ. *Int J Cancer.* 116(6):963-71. op cit.

Avon Breast Cancer Crusade
Available from: http://www.avoncompany.com/women/avoncrusade/index.html. Accessed August 17, 2005.

PART FIVE TAKING ACTION

18 Cancer registries

Cancer registries
Parkin DM, Whelan SL, Ferlay J, Teppo L and Thomas DB, editors. *IARC Scientific publication 155.* opcit.

Wow – cancer registries
Parkin DM. International variation. *Oncogene* 2004;23:6329-40.

Sir Richard Doll
Doll R, Payne P, Waterhouse JAH, editors. *Cancer Incidence in Five Continents, Vol I.* Geneva: Internationale Contre le Cancer; 1966; *Vol II*; 1970 op cit.

Membership of IACR
www.iacr.com.fr

Cancer statistics
Parkin DM, Whelan S, Ferlay J and Storm H. *Cancer Incidence in Five Continents*, *Vol I to VIII.* op cit.

19 Research

Quote
John E Fogarty International Center for

Advanced Study in Health Sciences. Justification. Available from: http://www.fic.nih.gov/about/2005cj.html. Accessed July 12, 2005.

Text
Magrath I. Grand Strategies – 1. The War on Cancer. *Network – The Newsletter of the International Network for Cancer Treatment and Research* 2003;4(1):1-6.

Cancer research spending by charities and government
Wows
Economic burden of cancer in Canada, 1998. Available from: http://www.cancer.ca/ccs/internet/standard/0,3182,3172_367655_37909904 8_langId-en,00.html. Accessed April 12, 2005.

Studies in the International Cancer Research Portfolio database
International Cancer Research Portfolio (ICRP). Available from: http://www.cancerportfolio.org.

Wow – Europe and USA, 2002-03 – prevention
European Cancer Research Managers Forum (ECRM). European Cancer Research Funding Survey March 2005. Available from: http://www.ecrmforum.org/report/ECRM_report.pdf. Accessed May 25, 2005.

Clinical trials
ClinicalTrials.gov. Available from: http://clinicaltrials.gov/ct/gui/search;jsessionid=1291B6E67BAB09F3560388ED5B4FA70D?term=cancer. Accessed May 13, 2005.

Study protocols of the European Organisation for Research and Treatment of Cancer (EORTC)
European Organisation for Research and Treatment of Cancer (EORTC). *EORTC protocols database – protocols by treatment.* Available from: http://www.eortc.be/protoc/listtrt.asp. Accessed July 13, 2005.

Funding in USA
National Institutes of Health (NIH). *NIH disease funding table – special areas of interest.* Available from: http://www.nih.gov/news/fundingresearchareas.htm. Accessed May 13, 2005.

20 Primary prevention

Text
Cancer Facts and Figures. op cit.
World Health Organization. *Cancer: diet and physical activity's impact.* Geneva: WHO. Available from: http://www.who.int/dietphysicalactivity/publications/facts/cancer/en. Accessed February 8, 2005.
Joint WHO/FAO expert consultation. *Diet, Nutrition, and Prevention of Chronic Diseases.* Geneva: WHO; 2003.

Immunization
World Health Organization. *World Health Report 2005 – Make Every Mother and Child Count.* Geneva: WHO; 2005.

Quit smoking
Thun MJ, Henley SJ, Calle EE: Tobacco use and cancer: an epidemiologic perspective for geneticists. *Oncogene* 2002;21:7307–25. [CPS (Cancer Prevention Study) is a cohort study of over a million participants in the USA. CPS II was launched in early 1980s by the American Cancer Society.]

Healthy consumer choices
Hawkes C. *Nutrition labels and health claims: the global regulatory environment.* Geneva: WHO; 2004.
Health, Welfare and Food Bureau, Government Logistics Department, Hong Kong Special Administrative Region, China. Consultation Paper on labelling scheme on nutrition information. November 2003;34.

Wow – Taiwan
Chang MH. Decreasing incidence of hepatocellular carcinoma among children following universal hepatitis B immunization. *Liver Int* 2003; 23:309–14.

21 Prevention: population and systems approaches

Quote
Available from: http://www.great-quotes.com.

Text
The Cancer Council Australia. *National Cancer Prevention Policy, 2004–06*. New South Wales: The Cancer Council Australia. Available from: http://www.cancer.org.au/documents/NCPP_full_contents_links.pdf.

McCarthy WH. The Australian experience in sun protection and screening for melanoma. *Journal of Surgical Oncology* 2004;86:236–45.

World Health Organization. *National cancer control programmes: policies and managerial guidelines*. 2nd ed. Geneva: WHO; 2002.

Effectiveness of measures to prevent smoking in young people
Farrelly MC, Davis KC, Haviland ML, Messeri P, Healton CG. Evidence of a dose-response relationship between "truth" anti-smoking ads and youth smoking prevalence. *Am J Public Health* 2005;95:425–31.

Miguel-Baquilod M, Fishburn B, Santos J, Jones NR, Warren CW: Tobacco use among students aged 13–15 years – Philippines, 2000 and 2003. *MMWR* 2005;54:94-97.

Shade structures
Wow – Victoria, Australia
The Cancer Council Victoria. *SunSmart Program 2003–06*. Victoria: The Cancer Council Victoria; 2002. Available from: http://www.sunsmart.com.au/downloads/about_sunsmart/sunsmart_program_2003_2006.pdf.

Cervical cancer prevention
Bray F, Loos AH, McCarron P, Weiderpass E, Arbyn M, Møller H, Hakama M, Parkin DM: Trends in cervical squamous cell carcinoma incidence in 13 European countries: changing risk and the effects of screening. *Cancer Epidemiology, Biomarkers & Prevention* 2005;14:677–86.

Bulk S, Visser O, Rozendaal L, Verheijen RHM, Meiher CJLM: Cervical cancer in the Netherlands 1989–1998: Decrease of squamous cell carcinoma in older women, increase of adenocarcinoma in younger women. *Int J Cancer* 2005;113:1005–09.

Number of physicians reported to be working in non-communicable disease control
Alwan A, Maclean D, Mandil A. *Assessment of national capacity for non-communicable disease prevention and control: the report of a global survey*. Geneva: WHO; 2001. Available from: http://whqlibdoc.who.int/hq/2001/WHO_MNC_01.2.pdf

22 Early detection

Quote
Available from: http://www.motivatingquotes.com/healthq.htm. Accessed April 12, 2005.

Text
World Health Organization. *National cancer control programmes: policies and managerial guidelines*. 2nd ed. Geneva: WHO; 2002.

Status of cervical cancer screening
International Agency for Research on Cancer. *IARC Handbooks of Cancer Prevention, Cervix Cancer Screening*. Geneva: WHO; 2005.

Anttila A, Ronco G, Clifford G, Bray F, Hakama M, et al. Cervical cancer screening programmes and policies in 18 European countries. *British Journal of Cancer* 2004; 91:935–41.

Aristotelous A. Cancer control programs in Cyprus – early detection and screening, personal communication, April 8, 2005, aaristotelous@ds.moh.gov.cy.

Bray F, Loos AH, McCarron P, Weiderpass E, Arbyn M, et al. *Cancer Epidemiology, Biomarkers & Prevention*. op cit.

Participation
Aristotelous A. op cit.

Fracheboud J. National Evaluation Team for Breast Cancer Screening (NETB) 2002 data, personal communication, March 17, 2005, j.fracheboud@erasmusmc.nl.

Patnick J, editor. *NHS Breast Screening Programme Annual Review 2003*. Sheffield: NHS Cancer Screening Programmes; 2003.

Lynge E, Olsen AH, Fracheboud J, Patnick J. Reporting of performance indicators of mammography screening in Europe. *European Journal of Cancer Prevention* 2003;12:213–22.

BreastScreen Aotearoa Independent Monitoring Group *Monitoring Report No 7*. Otago:University of Otago; 2001.

Australian Institute of Health and Welfare (AIHW). *BreastScreen Australia Monitoring Report 2001–2002, Cancer Series No 29*. Canberra:AIHW;2005.

Dean PB, Pamilo M. Screening mammography in Finland – 1.5 million examinations with 97 percent specificity. *Acta Oncologica Suppl* 1999;13:47–54.

Salas D. Valenica Breast Cancer Screening Programme – Spain (VBCSP) 2002 data, personal communication, March 9, 2005, salas_dol@gva.es.

Alberdi RZ. Programma Gallego de Detección Precoz del Cáncer de Mama, Galicia, Espana 2004 data, personal communication April 1, 2005, raquel.zubizarreta.alberdi@sergas.es.

Centre de dépistage du cancer du sein de la Ligue fribourgeoise contre le cancer. Rapport *d'activité 2004*.

Fondation pour le dépistage du cancer du sein. *Rapport d'activité 2003*.

Terzo Rapporto dell'Osservatorio Nasionale per la Prevenzione dei Tumori Femminili. *Rapporto Anno 2004*. Available from: http://www.osservatoriotumori.it/osservatorio/pubblicazioni/pubblicazioni.htm. Accessed April 1, 2005.

Hofvind SS-H, Wang J, Thoresen S. The Norwegian Breast Cancer Screening Program: re-attendance related to the women's experiences, intentions and previous screening result. *Cancer Causes and Control* 2003;14:391–98.

Olsen AH, Jensen A, Njor SH, Villadsen E, Schwartz W, et al.: Breast cancer incidence after the start of mammography screening in Denmark. *British Journal of Cancer* 2003;88:362–65.

Chiarelli A, Coldman A, Doyle G, Mah Z, Major D, Bancej C, Gomi A, Onysko J, Semenciw R, Wan G, editors. Organized breast cancer screening programmes in Canada, 1999 and 2000 report. Ottawa: Health Canada. Available from: http://www.phac-aspc.gc.ca/publicat/obscp-podcs00/index.html. Accessed March 2, 2005.

Swan J, Breen N, Coates RJ, Rimer BK, Lee NC. Progress in cancer screening practices in the United States. Results from the 2000 National Health Interview Survey. *Cancer* 2003;97:1528–40.

Public awareness

With permission from Keighley M, for the Public Affairs Committee, United European Gastroenterology Federation (UEGF). Raising awareness about colorectal screening in Europe. *CancerFutures* 2004;3:103–06.

Wow – screening

IARC Handbooks of Cancer Prevention, Cervix Cancer Screening. op cit.

23 Management and treatment

Quote

Accessed April 19, 2005 from http://www.motivatingquotes.com/healthq.htm.

Text

Getta G, Capocaccia R, Coleman MP, Gloeckler-Ries LA, Berrino F. Childhood cancer survival in Europe and the United States. *Cancer* 95:1767–72.

International Atomic Energy Agency. Millions of cancer victims in developing countries lack access to life-saving radiotherapy. November 2003. Accessed April 21, 2005 from http://www.iaea.org/NewsCenter/PressReleases/2003/prn0311.shtml.

International Atomic Energy Agency. *DIRAC – Directory of Radiotherapy Centers.* Vienna:IAEA;2000.

Availability of treatment

DIRAC – Directory of Radiotherapy Centers. op cit.

Zubizarreta EH, Poitevin A, Levin CV. Overview of radiotherapy resources in Latin America: a survey by the International Atomic Energy Agency

(IAEA). *Radiotherapy and Oncology* 2004;73:97–100.

United Nations Population Division. *World Population Prospects – The 2002 Revision.* Available from: http://www.un.org/esa/population/publications/wpp2002/wpp2002annextables.PDF. Accessed April 19, 2005.

Levin CV, Gueddari BE, Meghzifene A. Radiation therapy in Africa: distribution and equipment. *Radiotherapy and Oncology* 1999;52:79–84.

Tatsuzaki H, Levin CV. Quantitative status of resources for radiation therapy in Asia and Pacific region. *Radiotherapy and Oncology* 2001;60:81–89.

IAEA: DIRAC – Directory of Radiotherapy Centres. Accessed June 23, 2005 from: http://www-naweb.iaea.org/hanu/dirac/query3.asp

Parkin DM: Radiotherapy in Africa. Personal communication, June 22, 2005, ctsu0138@herald.ox.ac.uk

Wow – alternative medicine

Ernst E, Cassileth BR. The prevalence of complementary/alternative medicine in cancer – a systematic review. *Cancer* 1998; 83:777–82.

Richardson MA, Sanders T, Palmer JL, Greisinger A, Singletary SE. Complementary/alternative medicine use in a comprehensive cancer center and the implications for oncology. *Journal of Clinical Oncology* 2000;18:2505–2514.

White JD. Complementary and alternative medicine research: a National Cancer Institute perspective. *Semin Oncol* 2002;29:546–51.

Relative costs

International Atomic Energy Agency. *Programme of Action for Cancer Therapy.* Available from: http://www.iaea.org/NewsCenter/Features/Radiotherapy/gov2004-39_derestict.pdf. Accessed May 11, 2004.

Federal Trade Commission *Cigarette Report for 2002;* 2004. Available from: http://www.ftc.gov/reports/cigarette/041022cigaretterpt.pdf. Accessed April 26, 2005.

Trends in breast-cancer surgery

Edwards BK, Brown ML, Wingo PA, Howe HL, Ward E, et al. Annual report to the nation on the status of cancer, 1975–2002, featuring population-based trends in cancer treatment. *Journal of the National Cancer Institute 2005*; 97:1407-27.

24 Cancer organizations

Quote

Available from: http://www.quotationspage.com/quotes/William_Shakespeare.

Developing alliances and partnerships

Luis A Guillermo with the Venezuelan Cancer Society, personal communication, lguillermo@sociedadanticancerosa.org.

The Charter of Paris

UICC: http://www.uicc.org/index.php?id=1014. http://www.mychildmatters.org/

UICC World Cancer Congresses

Isabel Mortara, executive director of UICC, October 2004, personal communication.

Wow – UICC

Available from: http://www.uicc.org/index.php?id=482. Accessed August 19, 2005.

Wow – World Cancer Day

Available from: http://www.mychildmatters.org. Accessed August 19, 2005.

25 Health education

Quote

Available from: http://www.quotationspage.com/subjects/education/11.html. Accessed October 10, 2004.

World cancer days in 2005

Available from: http://www.cancer.org.au/content.cfm?randid=681715. Accessed April 24,

2005.
http://www.icccpo.org/. Accessed May 2
and 22, 2005.
http://www.who.int/tobacco/resources/
publications/wntd/2005/en/. Accessed
May 22, 2005.
http://www.qldcancer.com.au/Fundraisin
g/PinkRibbonDay.html. Accessed May
22, 2005.
http://www.bosombuddies.com.au/Field
_of_Women.htm. Accessed May 2, 2005.

26 Policies and legislation

Quote
Available from:
http://www.quotationspage.com/subjec
ts/laws/11.html. Accessed October 10,
2004.

Text
World Health Organization. National
cancer control programmes.
Geneva:WHO; 2002:115. Available
from:
http://www.who.int/cancer/media/en/
408.pdf. Accessed March 13, 2005.

WHO Framework Convention on Tobacco Control
Available from: http://www.who.int/en/.
Accessed December 1, 2004. NB:
Armenia and Nauru were not signatories
but acceded to the treaty, which has the
same effect as ratification.

Cancer programmes worldwide
World Health Organization. National
cancer control programmes. Geneva:
WHO 2002: table 10.1:115. Available
from:
http://www.who.int/cancer/media/en/
408.pdf. Accessed March 13, 2005.

Legislation
Alwan A, Maclean D, Mandil A. *Assessment
of national capacity for non-communicable
disease prevention and control: the report of a
global survey*. op cit.

PART SIX THE FUTURE & THE PAST

27 The future

Quote
Available from: http://www.aphids.com.
Accessed March 11, 2005.
http://www.worldofquotes.com/author
/Roger-Babson/1/. Accessed March 11,
2005.

Text
World Health Organization. International
Union Against Cancer. *Global Action
Against Cancer* 2003:6-8, 10-11; 2005.
Ferlay J, Bray F, Pisani P, Parkin DM. *IARC
CancerBase No 5*, version 2.0. op cit.

New cancer cases
IARC CancerBase No 5, version 2.0. op cit.

Cancer deaths
Global Action Against Cancer 2005. op cit.

Risk factors
Mackay J, Eriksen M. *The Tobacco Atlas*.
Geneva: WHO; 2002: p90–91.
Population Division of the Department of
Economic and Social Affairs of the United
Nations Secretariat. *World Population
Prospects: The 2004 Revision* and *World
Urbanization Prospects: The 2003 Revision*.
Available from: http://esa.un.org/unpp.
Accessed March 27, 2005.
International Association for the Study of
Obesity, and International Obesity Task
Force. *Projected Obesity Ranges in Europe,
2005–30*. May 2005.
International Food Information Council.
Food Insight. January/February 2001.

Action
Vaccine against cervical cancer : A vaccine
that may prevent cervical cancer could be
available within three years, UK experts
believe. Available from:
http://news.bbc.co.uk/go/em/-
/2/hi/health/3964263.stm. Accessed
October 29, 2004.
Unger JM, et al. Estimated impact of the
prostate cancer prevention trial on
population mortality. Cancer
2005;103(7):1375-80.

Hou HC. A scientific review of current
application of stem cell transplantation in
oncology. *Continuing Medical Education,
Medical Progress*. December 2003:45.
The Tobacco Atlas. op cit.
Pearson I. *Atlas of the Future*. New York:
Macmillan Books; 1998. p 32–33.
Cancer vaccine trial "promising". Scientists
develop a vaccine which may protect
people who have had cancer from
relapsing. Available from:
http://news.bbc.co.uk/go/em/-
/2/hi/health/3906703.stm. Accessed
July 19, 2004.
George Au, oncologist, Hong Kong,
personal communication, January 25,
2005.
American Federation for Aging Research.
What is the future of heart disease
research likely to tell us? Available from:
http://www.infoaging.org/d-heart-11-
future.html. Accessed January 3, 2004.
Crossman D. Science, medicine, and the
future. The future of the management of
ischaemic heart disease. *BMJ*
1997;314:356–59.
Guttmacher AE, Collins FS. Genomic
medicine: a primer. *N Engl J Med*
2002;347:1512–50.
Wolf CR, Smith G, Smith RL. Science,
medicine, and the future:
pharmacogenetics. *BMJ*
2000;320:987–90.
Kampe B. Symposium reveals future of
cancer. Distinguished panel presents
progress of preventative medicines.
Available from:
http://www.dailybruin.ucla.edu/news/a
rticles.asp?id=30790. Accessed January
23, 2005.
Roden DM. Cardiovascular
pharmacogenomics. *Circulation*
2003;108:3071–3074.

The history of cancer

Major sources
Cancer Council of Victoria. Timeline –
cancer through history. Available from:
http://www.cancervic.org.au/cancer1/s
tudents/cancer_history.htm.
Lane S. Rare Cancer Alliance. Cancer
History, 2004. Available from:
http: www.rare-cancer.org/history-of-

cancer.html.

Lee HSJ, Wright J, *Dates in Oncology: A Chronological Record of Progress in Oncology over the Last Millennium*. Taylor & Francis Group, 2000.

Notes from cancer: a narrative exploration. Session 1: an ancient enemy? Available from: http://www.thestupidschool.ca/fgp/Projects/cancer/cane-1.htm.

American Cancer Society, The history of cancer. Available from: http://www.cancer.org/docroot/CRI/content/CRI_2_6x_the_history_of_cancer_72.asp?sitearea=CRI.

History of cancer treatments. Available from: http://student.biology.arizona.edu/honors2002/group07/hist.html.

Cohen I, Tagliaferri M, Tripathy LA and D. *Journal of Chinese Medicine* No 68, February 2002. Part One: Traditional Chinese medicine in the treatment of breast cancer. Available from: http://www.cancerlynx.com/chinesemedicine.html.

Tobacco facts. From first drag to slavery: tobacco's beginnings (to the late 19th century). Available from: http://www.tobaccofacts.org/tob_truth/timeline1492.html.

National Cancer Institute. Closing in on cancer – solving a 5000-year mystery. Available from: http://rex.nci.nih.gov/behindthenews/cioc/contents/contents.htm.

Freireich EJ. Min Chiu Li: a perspective in cancer therapy. *Clinical Cancer Research* September 2002;8:2764–65.

Cell biology and cancer. Available from: http://science.education.nih.gov/supplements/nih1/cancer/guide/intro1.htm.

Lyons AS, Petrucelli RJ II. *Medicine: An Illustrated History*. New York: Harry N Abrams Inc; 1978. p 587.

http://www.nobelprize.org

PART SEVEN WORLD TABLES

Part-title quote

http://www.quotationspage.com/quotes/Julia_Child/

Table A Risk factors for cancer

1 Population

http://www.who.int

UN Population and Vital Statistics Report: Series A, Table 2. Population, latest available census and estimates for 2002 or 2003. Available online at: http://unstats.un.org/unsd/demographic/products/vitstats/seriesa2.htm. Accessed Sept 30, 2005.

2 Youth smoking prevalence

See sources above for **3 Risk for boys, Early starters**

3 Adult smoking prevalence

See sources above for **5 Tobacco, Smoking among adults**

4 Overweight prevalence

See sources above for **7 Diet and nutrition, Overweight**

Table B Statistics on cancer

1 The risk of getting cancer

See sources above for **10 The risk of getting cancer, Cancer risk**

2 Cancer survivors

See sources above for **15 Cancer survivors, Five-year cancer survivors**

3 Primary prevention

See sources above for **20 Primary prevention, Immunization**

4 Incidence of cancer

See sources above for **12 Geographical diversity, Incidence of cancer** *and* **13 Lung cancer, Lung cancer incidence**

WHO HQ and Regional Offices

WHO HQ, Switzerland
http://www.who.int/
 WHO RO Africa (AFRO), Congo
http://www.afro.who.int/
 WHO RO Americas/PAHO (PAHO/AMRO), USA
http://www.paho.org/
 WHO RO Eastern Mediterranean (EMRO), Egypt
http://www.emro.who.int/
 WHO RO Europe (EURO), Denmark
http://www.euro.who.int/
 WHO RO South-East Asia (SEARO), India
Main: http://w3.whosea.org/
 WHO RO Western Pacific (WPRO), Philippines
http://www.wpro.who.int/

WHO Cancer Programmes

International Agency for Research on Cancer (IARC), France:
 http://www.iarc.fr/
Database: http://www-dep.iarc.fr/dataava/infodata.htm
WHO Cancer programmes, Switzerland:
 http://www.who.int/cancer/en/

Cancer Organizations by Country

Argentina
Liga Argentina de Lucha Contra el Cáncer:
 http://www.lalcecsanisidro.org.ar/Obrasyservicios.html
Australia
National Cancer Control Initiative:
 http://www.ncci.org.au/index.htm
Peter MacCallum Cancer Institute: http://www.petermac.org/
Queensland Cancer Fund: http://www.qldcancer.com.au/
The Cancer Council ACT: http://www.actcancer.org/
The Cancer Council Australia: http://www.cancer.org.au/
The Cancer Council New South Wales:
 http://www.cancercouncil.com.au/
The Cancer Council Northern Territory:
 http://www.cancercouncilnt.com.au/
The Cancer Council South Australia:
 http://www.cancersa.org.au/
The Cancer Council Tasmania: http://www.cancertas.org.au/
The Cancer Council Victoria:
 http://www.cancervic.org.au/index.htm
The Cancer Council Western Australia:
 http://www.cancerwa.asn.au/
Walter and Eliza Hall Institute of Medical Research:
 http://www.wehi.edu.au/
Austria
Austrian Cancer Society: http://www.krebshilfe.net/home.shtm
Bahrain
Bahrain Cancer Society
Bangladesh
Bangladesh Cancer Society
Belgium
Association of European Cancer Leagues: http://ecl.uicc.org/
Belgian Federation against Cancer: http://www.cancer.be/
European Oncology Nursing Society:
 http://www.cancerworld.org/CancerWorld/moduleStatic

Page.aspx?id=1275&id_sito=2&id_stato=1
European Organisation for Research and Treatment of Cancer:
 http://www.eortc.be/
European Society of Surgical Oncology: http://www.esso-surgeonline.be/
European Society for Therapeutic Radiation and Oncology:
 http://www.estro.be/
Federation of European Cancer Societies:
 http://www.fecs.be/emc.asp
Flemish League Against Cancer: http://www.tegenkanker.net/
International Network for Cancer Treatment and Research:
 http://www.inctr.org/
Oncologic Center Antwerp:
 http://www.wijook.be/ocasite/index.htm
Bolivia
Fundación Boliviana Contra el Cáncer
Brazil
Fundação Oncocentro de Sao Paulo:
 http://www.fosp.saude.sp.gov.br/
Instituto Brasileiro de Contrôle do Câncer:
 http://www.ibcc.org.br/
Instituto Nacional do Cancer: http://www.inca.gov.br/
Liga Bahiana Contra o Cancer:
 http://www.aristidesmaltez.org.br/
Sociedade Brasileira de Cancerologia:
 http://www.sbcancer.org.br/
Cameroon
African Organisation for Research and Training in Cancer
 http://www.aortic.org/
Canada
British Columbia Cancer Agency: http://www.bccancer.bc.ca/
Canadian Cancer Society/National Cancer Institute of Canada:
 http://www.cancer.ca/ccs/
Cancer Care Ontario: http://www.cancercare.on.ca/
Centre for Chronic Disease and Prevention: http://www.hc-sc.gc.ca/
Fondation Québécoise du Cancer: http://www.fqc.qc.ca/
Princess Margaret Hospital: http://www.uhnres.utoronto.ca/
China
Chinese Anti-Cancer Association: http://www.caca.org.cn/
Chinese Medical Association - Beijing:
 http://www.chinamed.com.cn/
Hong Kong Anti-Cancer Society: http://www.hkacs.org.hk/
Tianjin Medical University Cancer Institute and Hospital:
 http://www.tjmuch.com/
Formosa Cancer Foundation: http://www.fcf.org.tw/
John Tung Foundation: http://www.jtf.org.tw/JTF01/01-04.asp
Colombia
Liga Colombiana Contra el Cáncer:
 http://www.ligacancercolombia.org/
Croatia
Croatian League Against Cancer
Cuba
Instituto Nacional de Oncología y Radiobiología
Cyprus
Cyprus Anti-Cancer Society:
 http://www.anticancersociety.org.cy
Cyprus Association of Cancer Patients and Friends:
 http://www.cancercare.org.cy/EN/index.html
Czech Republic
League Against Cancer Prague: http://www.lpr.cz/

Denmark
Danish Cancer Society: http://www.cancer.dk/
Faroese Association against Cancer: http://www.krabbamein.fo/
Dominican Republic
Liga Dominicana Contra el Cáncer
Patronato Cibaeño Contra el Cáncer
Ecuador
Sociedad de Lucha contra el Cáncer: http://www.solca.med.ec/
Egypt
National Cancer Institute, Cairo: http://www.nci.edu.eg/
African Organisation for Research and Training in Cancer
   http://www.aortic.org/
El Salvador
Instituto del Cáncer de El Salvador
Estonia
Estonian Cancer Society:
   http://www.cancer.ee/?op=&id=&cid=
Fiji
Fiji Cancer Society
Finland
Association of Nordic Cancer Registries:
   http://ncu.cancer.dk/ancr/default.shtml
Cancer Society of Finland: http://www.cancer.fi/
France
Centre d'Oncologie Léon Bérard: http://oncora1.lyon.fnclcc.fr/
Centre Régional François Baclesse: http://www.cgfl.com/
Centre Régional Jean Perrin: http://www.cjp.fr/
Centre René Gauducheau: http://www.valdorel.fnclcc.fr/
Epidaure C.R.L.C. Val d'Aurelle-Paul Lamarque:
   http://www.valdorel.fnclcc.fr/
European Network of Cancer Registries:
   http://www.encr.com.fr/
Fédération Nationale des Centres de Lutte contre le Cancer:
   http://www.fnclcc.fr/
Institut Claudius Regaud: http://www.claudiusregaud.fr/
Institut Curie: http://www.curie.fr/
Institut Gustave Roussy: http://www.igr.fr/
Institut Paoli Calmettes: http://www.institutpaolicalmettes.fr/
International Association of Cancer Registries:
   http://www.iacr.com.fr/
Ligue Nationale Comité de Paris: http://www.lvc.ch/
Ligue Nationale Contre le Cancer: http://www.ligue-cancer.net/
Georgia
National Cancer Centre of Georgia
Germany
Deutsches Krebsforschungszentrum: http://www.dkfz.de/
Deutsche Krebsgesellschaft e.V:
   http://www.krebsgesellschaft.de/
Deutsche Krebshilfe: http://www.krebshilfe.de/
European Association for Neuroncology: http://www.eano.de/
Greece
Hellenic Cancer Society: http://www.cancer-society.gr/
Guatemala
Liga Nacional Contra el Cáncer Guatemala/Piensa
Honduras
Associación Hondureña de Lucha Contra el Cáncer
Liga Contra el Cáncer
Hungary
Hungarian League Against Cancer: http://www.rakliga.hu/
Iceland
Icelandic Cancer Society: http://www.krabb.is/

India
Bangalore Institute of Oncology: http://www.biohospital.org/
Cancer Centre Welfare Home and Research Institute:
   http://www.cancercentrecalcutta.org/
Cancer Patients Aid Association: http://www.cpaaindia.org/
Dharamshila Cancer Hospital: http://www.cancerdch.org/
Dr. B. Borooah Cancer Institute: http://www.bbci-gau.org/
Gujarat Cancer and Research Institute:
   http://www.cancerindia.org/
Indian Cancer Society: http://www.indiancancersociety.org/
Institute of Cytology and Preventive Oncology:
   http://icmr.nic.in/pinstitute/icpo.htm
Kidwai Memorial Institute of Oncology:
   http://kar.nic.in/kidwai/
Rajiv Gandhi Cancer Institute and Research Centre:
   http://www.rgci.com/
Regional Cancer Centre, Thiruvananthapuram:
   http://www.rcctvm.org/
Tata Memorial Centre: http://www.tatamemorialcentre.com/
Indonesia
Indonesian Cancer Foundation
Iran
Cancer Institute, Imam Khomeini Medical Center:
   http://www.health-net.or.jp/kenkonet/tobacco/front.html
Ireland
Irish Cancer Society: http://www.cancer.ie/
Israel
Israel Cancer Association: http://www.cancer.org.il/home.asp
Middle East Cancer Consortium: http://mecc.cancer.gov/
Italy
Associazione Italiana di Oncologia Medica: http://www.aiom.it/
Associazione Italiana Malati di Cancro Parenti e Amici:
   http://www.aimac.it/
Associazione Italiana per la Ricerca sul Cancro:
   http://www.airc.it/
Centro di Riferimento Oncologico:
   http://www.cro.sanita.fvg.it/
Centro per lo Studio E la Prevenzione Oncologica:
   http://www.cspo.it/
European Institute of Oncology:
   http://www.ieo.it/italiano/index.htm
European School of Oncology:
   http://www.cancerworld.org/cancerworld/home.aspx?id_sito
   =1&id_stato=1
Fondazione 'G. Pascale': http://www.fondazionepascale.it/
IST Istituto Nazionale per la Ricerca sul Cancro:
   http://www.istge.it/
Istituto di Ricerche Farmacologiche 'Mario Negri':
   http://www.marionegri.it/
Istituto Nazionale per lo Studio e la Cura dei Tumori:
   http://www.istitutotumori.mi.it/int/default.asp
Istituto Oncologico Romagnolo: http://www.ior-forli.it/
Lega Italiana per la Lotta Contro I Tumori:
   http://www.legatumori.it/
Regina Elena Cancer Institute: http://crs.ifo.it/
Università degli Studi dell' Insubria:
   http://www3.uninsubria.it/uninsubria/home.html
Università degli Studi di Perugia: http://www.unipg.it/
Japan
Aichi Cancer Center:
   http://www.pref.aichi.jp/cancercenter/english/overview/gan.html

The Asian Pacific Organization for Cancer Prevention:
  http://www.apocp.org/
Cancer Institute of JFCR: http://www.jfcr.or.jp/
Chiba Cancer Center:
  http://www.pref.chiba.jp/byouin/gan/en/
Children's Cancer Association of Japan: http://www.ccaj-found.or.jp/
Hokkaido Cancer Society: http://www.sapmed.ac.jp/
Japan Cancer Society: http://www.jcancer.jp/eng/
Japan Society of Clinical Oncology: http://jsco.umin.ac.jp/
Japanese Cancer Association: http://www.jca.gr.jp/
Kanagawa Cancer Center:
  http://www.pref.kanagawa.jp/osirase/byouin/gan/index.htm
Osaka Medical Center for Cancer and Cardiovascular Diseases:
  http://www.mc.pref.osaka.jp/
Princess Takamatsu Cancer Research Fund:
  http://www.ptcrf.or.jp/
Saitama Cancer Center:
  http://www.pref.saitama.jp/A80/BA02/top-e.htm
Sapporo Cancer Seminar Foundation: http://www.phoenix-c.or.jp/scs-hk/
Science Council of Japan:
  http://www.scj.go.jp/en/scj/about/index.html
Tochigi Cancer Center: http://www.tcc.pref.tochigi.jp/
Jordan
King Hussein Cancer Center: www.khcc.jo
Kenya
Kenya Cancer Association
Kuwait
Kuwait Society for Smoking and Cancer Prevention
Latvia
August Kirchenstein Institute of Microbiology and Virology:
  http://www.micro.lv/
Lebanon
Lebanese Cancer Society: http://www.cancer.org.lb/
Lithuania
Lithuanian Anti-Cancer Association
Luxembourg
Fondation Luxembourgeoise: http://www.cancer.lu/
Malaysia
Asia-Pacific Hospice Palliative Care Network:
  http://www.aphn.org/Index.asp
Cancer Society of Sabah: http://www.sabah.org.my/scss/cancer/
MAKNA-National Cancer Council:
  http://www.makna.org.my/index.aspx
National Cancer Society of Malaysia: http://www.cancer.org.my/
Mexico
Instituto Nacional de Cancerología - México:
  http://www.incan.edu.mx/
Sociedad Mexicana de Estudios Oncológicos AC:
  http://www.smeo.org.mx/
Mongolia
National Oncological Centre - Mongolia
Namibia
Cancer Association of Namibia: http://www.can.org.na/
Nepal
BP Koirala Memorial Cancer Hospital:
  http://www.yomari.com/bpkmch/contact.html
Nepal Cancer Relief Society: http://www.ncrs.org.np/
Netherlands
Academisch Medisch Centrum: http://www.amc.uva.nl/
Bone Marrow Donors Worldwide: http://www.bmdw.org/

Dutch Association of Comprehensive Cancer Centers:
  http://www.ikcnet.nl/IKN/nieuws/index.php
Dutch Cancer Society: http://www.kwfkankerbestrijding.nl/
European Cancer Centre: http://www.eurcancen.org/
European Cancer Patient Coalition: http://www.ecpc-online.org/resources.html
European Group for Blood and Marrow Transplantation:
  http://www.ebmt.org/
International Confederation of Childhood Cancer Parent
  Organisations:
  http://www.icccpo.org/
Netherlands Cancer Institute: http://www.nki.nl/
New Zealand
Cancer Society of New Zealand, Inc:
  http://www.cancernz.org.nz/
Nigeria
Nigerian Cancer Society
Norway
Norwegian Cancer Society:
  http://www.kreftforeningen.no/dt_front.asp?gid=317
Pakistan
Pakistan Atomic Energy Commission:
  http://www.paec.gov.pk/paec-ct.htm
Panama
Asociación Nacional Contra el Cáncer:
  http://www.panamatravel.com/ancec/mainanc.htm
Peru
Instituto de Enfermedades Neoplásicas: http://www.inen.sld.pe/
Liga Peruana de Lucha Contra el Cáncer:
  http://www.terra.com.pe:95/ligacancer/
Oncosalud SAC: http://www.oncosalud.com.pe/
Sociedad Peruana de Cancerología:
  http://www.spcancerologia.org/
Sociedad Peruana de Oncología Médica:
  http://www.spom.org.pe/
Philippines
Philippine Cancer Society: http://www.philcancer.org/
Poland
International Hereditary Cancer Center:
  http://www.hereditarycancer.net/eng/
Portugal
Instituto Português de Oncologia de Francisco Gentil:
  http://www.ipolisboa.min-saude.pt/
Liga Portuguesa Contra o Cancro:
  http://www.ligacontracancro.pt/
Republic of Korea
Republic of Korea Cancer Society: http://www.kirams.re.kr/
Republic of Korea National Cancer Center Research Institute:
  http://www.ncc.re.kr/
Romania
Institute of Oncology 'Al Trestioreanu' Bucharest
Russian Federation
N N Blokhin Cancer Research Center
N N Petrov Research Institute of Oncology
Saudi Arabia
Gulf Center for Cancer Registration:
  http://www.gccr.org/main.html
Serbia and Montenegro
Serbian Society for the Fight Against Cancer:
  http://www.serbiancancer.org/
Singapore
National Cancer Center - Singapore: http://www.nccs.com.sg/

Singapore Cancer Society:
http://www.singaporecancersociety.org.sg/

Slovakia
Slovak League Against Cancer: http://www.cancerfonden.se/

Slovenia
Institute of Oncology Ljubljana: http://www.onko-i.si/

South Africa
Cancer Association of South Africa: http://www.cansa.org.za/
African Organisation for Research and Training in Cancer
http://www.aortic.org/

Spain
Asociación Española Contra el Cáncer:
http://www.todocancer.com/esp
Asociación Vivir Como Antes
Institut Català d'Oncologia: http://www.iconcologia.net/

Sweden
Swedish Cancer Society: http://www.cancerfonden.se/

Switzerland
European Society for Medical Oncology: http://www.esmo.org/
Globalink: http://www.globalink.org/
International Union Against Cancer: http://www.uicc.org/
International Extranodal Lymphoma Study Group:
http://www.ielsg.org/
Krebsliga Schweiz: http://www.swisscancer.ch/
Ludwig Institute for Cancer Research: http://www.licr.org/

Syria
Syrian Cancer Society: http://www.scts-sy.org/

Thailand
National Cancer Institute - Thailand: http://www.nci.go.th/

Trinidad and Tobago
Trinidad and Tobago Cancer Society

Tunisia
Association Tunisienne de Lutte contre le Cancer:
http://www.atcc.org.tn/

Turkey
Turkish Association for Cancer Research and Control:
http://www.turkcancer.org/

Uganda (and UK)
Hospice Africa: http://hospice-africa.merseyside.org/

UK
British Association for Cancer Research:
http://www.bacr.org.uk/
British Association of Surgical Oncology:
http://www.baso.org.uk/index.html
Cancer Research UK: http://www.cancerresearchuk.org/
CancerBACUP: http://www.cancerbacup.org.uk/Home
Cochrane Cancer Network: http://www.canet.org/
European Association for Cancer Research:
http://www.eacr.org/
Guide to Internet Resources for Cancer:
http://www.cancerindex.org/clinks1.htm
Imperial Cancer Research Fund:
http://www.imperialcancer.co.uk/
International Ostomy Association:
http://www.ostomyinternational.org/
Ludwig Institute for Cancer Research: http://www.licr.org/
Macmillan Cancer Relief: http://www.macmillan.org.uk/
Marie Curie Cancer Care: http://www.mariecurie.org.uk/
Tenovus: http://www.tenovus.com/
The Institute of Cancer Research: http://www.icr.ac.uk/
The Paterson Institute for Cancer Research:

http://www.paterson.man.ac.uk/
Ulster Cancer Foundation: http://www.ulstercancer.org/
World Cancer Research Fund International:
http://www.wcrf.org/

Uruguay
Comisión Honoraria de Lucha Contra el Cáncer:
http://www.urucan.org.uy/
Hospital de Clínicas Dr. Manuel Quintela:
http://www.oncologiamedica.hc.edu.uy/

USA
American Association for Cancer Research:
http://www.aacr.org/
American Cancer Society: http://www.cancer.org
American College of Radiology:
http://www.acr.org/s_acr/index.asp
American College of Surgeons Commission on Cancer:
http://www.facs.org/cancer/index.html
American Society of Clinical Oncology: http://www.asco.org
American Society for Therapeutic Radiology and Oncology
(ASTRO): http://www.astro.org/
Association of Cancer Online Resources: http://www.acor.org/
C-Change (National Dialogue on Cancer): http://www.c-changetogether.org/
Centers for Disease Control and Prevention:
http://www.cdc.gov/cancer/
College of American Pathologists:
http://www.cap.org/apps/cap.portal
International Bone Marrow Transplant Registry:
http://www.ibmtr.org/
International Cancer Alliance for Research and Education:
http://www.icare.org/
International Relay For Life:
http://www.cancer.org/international.
International Society for the Study of Comparative Oncology:
http://www.iiar-anticancer.org/issco/issco_index.htm
Lance Armstrong Foundation: http://www.laf.org/
National Cancer Institute: http://www.cancer.gov
National Center for Tobacco-Free Kids:
http://www.tobaccofreekids.org/
North American Association of Central Cancer Registries:
http://www.naaccr.org/
Oncology Nursing Society: http://www.ons.org/
Society of Surgical Oncology Inc.: http://www.surgonc.org/

Venezuela
Sociedad Anticancerosa de Venezuela:
http://www.sociedadanticancerosa.org/PAGINAMARCOS.HTM

Viet Nam
National Cancer Institute – Viet Nam: http://www.nci.org.vn/

Zimbabwe
Cancer Association of Zimbabwe

INDEX